Fifth Edition
VETERINARY CLINICAL PARASITOLOGY

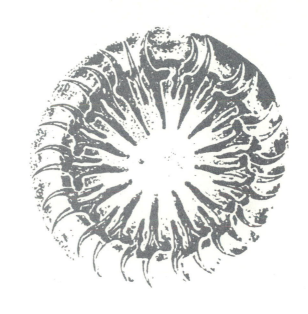

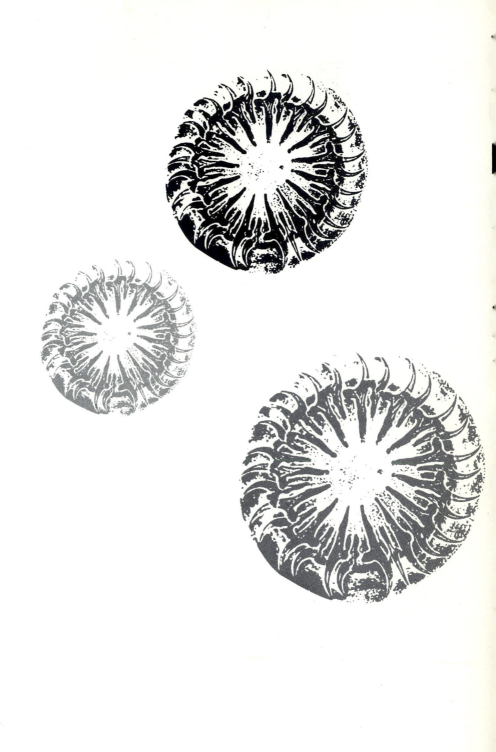

Fifth Edition

VETERINARY CLINICAL PARASITOLOGY

Margaret W. Sloss B.S., M.S., D.V.M.
Russell L. Kemp A.B., PH.D.

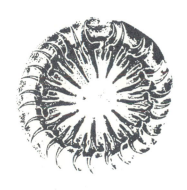

Iowa State University Press, Ames, Iowa

MARGARET W. SLOSS is professor emeritus of Veterinary Pathology and Parasitology at Iowa State University. She was in charge of the Veterinary Clinical Pathology Laboratory at Iowa State from its inception in 1938, the year she received her D.V.M. degree from that institution. She holds the B.S. degree in zoology and the M.S. in microscopic anatomy from Iowa State. Dr. Sloss is a past national president of the Women's Veterinary Medical Association and of Sigma Delta Epsilon and past president of Phi Kappa Phi and Phi Zeta honor societies at Iowa State. She is a member of the American Veterinary Medical Association, the Iowa Veterinary Medical Association, the American Association of Veterinary Parasitologists, the Veterinary Clinical Pathologists, and the Women's Veterinary Medical Association. She appears in *American Men of Science* 8th ed. (1949), *Who's Who of American Women,* 5th ed. (1968-69, 1970), *World Who's Who of Women,* 2nd ed. (1974-75) and *Notable Americans of the Bicentennial Era,* Vol. 1 (1976).

RUSSELL L. KEMP is professor of Veterinary Pathology and Parasitology at Iowa State University. He has been in charge of the teaching laboratory in Veterinary Parasitology since 1967, the year he joined the faculty. Dr. Kemp holds the A.B. degree from the College of Wooster, Wooster, Ohio, with emphasis on zoology, and the Ph.D. degree from the University of Georgia in poultry parasitology. He is a member of the honor societies of Sigma Xi, Phi Kappa Phi, Gamma Sigma Delta, and Phi Zeta. He is a member also of the American Society of Parasitologists, the Society of Protozoologists, and an associate member of the American Association of Avian Pathologists.

© 1978 Iowa State University Press, Ames, Iowa 50010
All rights reserved

Composed by Iowa State University Press
Printed in the United States of America

First, second, and third editions, 1948, 1955, by Edward A. Benbrook and Margaret W. Sloss; fourth edition, 1970, by Margaret W. Sloss.

Fifth edition, 1978
Second printing, 1979
Third printing, 1982
Fourth printing, 1984
Fifth printing, 1984
Sixth printing, 1985
Seventh printing, 1986

Library of Congress Cataloging in Publication Data

Sloss, Margaret Wragg, 1901-
    Veterinary clinical parasitology.

    Bibliography: p.
    Includes index.
    1. Veterinary parasitology. 2. Veterinary medicine — Diagnosis. I. Kemp, Russell L., joint author. II. Title. [DNLM: 1. Parasitic diseases — Veterinary — Lab manuals. 2. Parasitology — Laboratory manuals. SF810 S634v]
SF810.A3S58 1978   636.089′69′6   77-20156
ISBN 0-8138-1730-7

CONTENTS

PREFACE

The control of disease is successful only when preceded by accurate diagnosis. The basic diagnostic methods include (1) history, (2) clinical signs, (3) gross lesions, and (4) laboratory procedures. If an accurate diagnosis cannot be obtained by the first three methods, laboratory procedures are used for what assistance they may offer.

The purpose of this book is to assist in the diagnosis of various clinical and nonclinical parasitisms by means of laboratory methods. It is not intended to present life cycles and treatments in the manner of a textbook in parasitology. It is assumed that persons using this manual have had basic training in parasitology; therefore, the manual includes sufficient information to make it of practical value to students and graduates in veterinary medicine and laboratory animal medicine, to laboratory diagnosticians, and to others with a medical or zoological background who have occasion to deal with parasitisms in their work with animals.

Techniques and diagnostic findings are illustrated by means of original photomicrographs, gross photographs, and drawings. The publication is divided into five sections: (1) Fecal Examinations in the Diagnosis of Parasitism, (2) Parasites of the Blood, (3) Mites and Ticks (Acarina) of the Skin and Internal Organs, (4) Louse and Flea Infestations, (5) Miscellaneous Skin Parasites. The techniques presented are not necessarily the only usable ones but were selected on the basis of simplicity and proved effectiveness over many years and many thousands of cases.

Margaret W. Sloss
Russell L. Kemp

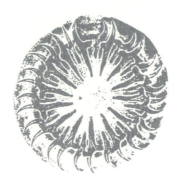

Section One

FECAL EXAMINATION IN THE DIAGNOSIS OF PARASITISM

Parasites inhabiting the digestive canal and biliary and urinary systems produce eggs, larvae, or cysts that leave the body of the host by way of the feces or urine. Occasionally even adult parasites may be seen in feces, especially when the host has enteritis. Parasitic worm eggs or larvae from the lower respiratory system are usually coughed into the pharynx and swallowed, and they too appear in feces (see Figs. 1.39, 1.65, 1.91, 1.105, 1.127, 1.200).

Many parasitic forms seen in feces have characteristic morphology that is diagnostic for a particular species of parasite (e.g., Figs. 1.17, 1.21, 1.67, 1.83, 1.107, 1.200). On the other hand, certain worm parasites produce eggs that may be recognized as those of nematodes, flukes, or tapeworms but cannot easily be separated as to the exact species of origin.

Mange or scab mites may be licked or nibbled from the skin, thus accounting for their appearance in the feces (see Fig. 1.142). Fecal examination may also reveal to a limited extent the status of digestion, as shown by the presence of undigested muscle (see Figs. 1.155, 1.156), starch, or fat droplets.

1

Animals may swallow certain objects that resemble parasite forms. These are known as *pseudoparasites;* they include such things as pollen grains, plant hairs, grain mites, mold spores, and a variety of harmless plant and animal debris (see Figs. 1.144–1.150, 1.153, 1.154, 1.181, 1.182, 1.209, 1.210). *Spurious parasites* are sometimes encountered in feces. For example, parasite eggs or cysts from one species of host may be found in the feces of a scavenger or predator host as the result of coprophagy (see Figs. 1.143, 1.151, 1.152).

COLLECTION OF FECAL SAMPLES

Fresh feces should be used whenever obtainable. Old samples may become dehydrated, making suspension difficult; also worm eggs or coccidial oocysts may undergo development, hatching, or disintegration to such a degree as to interfere with diagnosis.

Animal owners may submit fecal samples in all sorts of containers, suitable or not suitable. It is suggested that clients be supplied with clean, wide-mouthed, screw-capped or stoppered jars of at least 60 ml (2 oz) capacity. One or two wooden tongue depressors are convenient for picking up samples, after which they are discarded. Formed droppings may be transported for a few hours when well wrapped in waterproofed paper, foil, or plastic wrap.

At least several grams of feces should be collected for an examination. Because of the roughage content, larger samples should be secured from herbivorous than from carnivorous animals.

If defecation does not provide sufficient material, a sample may be taken directly from the rectum, or defecation may be induced quickly by inserting a suppository made from bar soap or a paper match from an ordinary match folder. Plain water enema samples may be obtained, but the dilution factor usually makes them undesirable. *Soapy or oily enemas should not be used.* Fecal specimens removed from rectal thermometers are seldom satisfactory in quantity.

If fecal material is to be transported for more than a few hours, it must be preserved. A 10% formaldehyde solution may be added to saturate the sample. Refrigeration will also keep samples in good condition for several days.

Fecal samples to be shipped by postal service, express, or other means should be enclosed in leak-proof containers. Proper identification of each sample by means of a label or a tag is necessary.

GROSS EXAMINATION

Gross examination should always be made for the detection of living or dead worms or for the detection of the segments of tapeworms. Oily or soapy substances in samples will indicate that microscopic examination will be difficult or even impossible.

CALIBRATION OF THE MICROSCOPE

Accurate identification of parasite eggs and cysts in fecal samples may require measurement. In order to accomplish this, a micrometer disk, such as shown in Figure 1.1, must be inserted into the ocular of the microscope and calibrated against a known reference in the form of a stage micrometer (Fig. 1.2). Each objective lens of the microscope must be individually calibrated with the ocular lens/micrometer combination to be used. The calibration will be accurate only for that particular microscope ocular and objective combination.

Calibration of the ×45 objective will illustrate the procedure for all lenses of the microscope to be calibrated. Place the stage micrometer on the stage of the microscope and focus until the lines are sharp. It may be necessary to adjust the condenser iris diaphragm for maximum contrast. In the example, the stage micrometer is 1 mm (1000 μm) long and is divided into 100 parts, thus each small division of the stage micrometer represents 10 μm. Superimpose any convenient numbered line of the ocular micrometer (usually the 0 mark) on a convenient line of the stage micrometer (the first large line in the example). The field should now resemble Figure 1.3. Find the two lines that are exactly superimposed. In the example, line 49 of the ocular micrometer falls exactly on line 11 of the stage micrometer. Thus 49 divisions of the unknown ocular micrometer represent 11 divisions, each of 10 μm length, or a total of 110 μm. (With some ocular/stage micrometer combinations a series of lines may correspond, but this makes no difference in the calibration procedure; any convenient pair may be chosen to continue the process.) To complete the calibration, divide 110 μm by 49 divisions, resulting in a calibration factor of 2.24 μm per division for the ocular micrometer in the example. Repeat this procedure for each objective lens to be calibrated on the microscope.

To use the calibrated microscope, superimpose the ocular micrometer scale on an egg or cyst and count the number of divi-

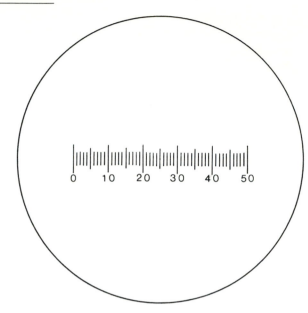

FIG. 1.1. A typical ocular micrometer of 50 divisions. The divisions have no meaning until calibrated against a stage micrometer.

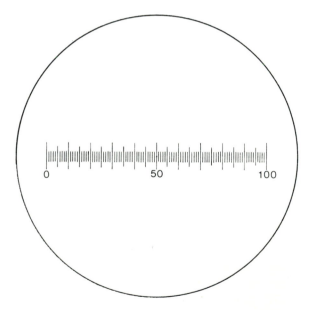

FIG. 1.2. A typical stage micrometer of 1 mm total length. Each division represents 10 μm.

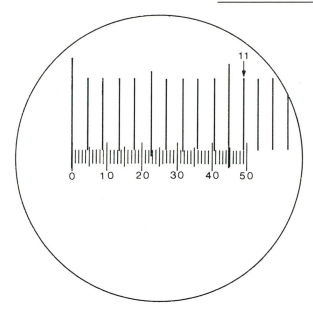

FIG. 1.3. Appearance at ×45 of an ocular micrometer being calibrated with a 10 microns/division stage micrometer. Note conjunction of line 11 of stage micrometer with line 49 of ocular micrometer.

sions subtended by the specimen, for example 12. Multiply 12 by the calibration factor (2.24 for the ×45 lens in the example); 12 x 2.24 = 26.88 μm, the size of the object being measured.

MICROSCOPIC EXAMINATION

Many techniques for microscopic examination have been published, and it is difficult to select one or two methods most useful for a veterinary clinical laboratory. Three qualitative techniques will be described in considerable detail, along with a brief appraisal of quantitative methods and reference to a commercially available system.

SIMPLE SMEAR TECHNIQUE

The simple smear technique is better than no examination at all, but it has many disadvantages. It should be used only when very small samples are available or when lack of equipment or time prevents the use of a more accurate technique. The procedure is as follows:

1. Place a microslide on a small piece of newspaper (regular reading matter).
2. Place a drop of tap water on the center of the slide.
3. With a toothpick or similar instrument, detach from the fecal mass a small sample, about 3 mm in diameter.
4. Mix the sample into the drop of water on the slide until the suspension is cloudy but not so much that the newsprint cannot be read through it. By means of a finely pointed forceps, remove any larger bits of debris that may be present.
5. Gently lower a square 18 mm or 22 mm glass or plastic coverglass onto the specimen on the microslide.
6. Examine systematically under low magnification ($\times 100$) of the microscope, using the high, dry magnification ($\times 400$) for observation of details (see Fig. 1.14).

QUALITATIVE CONCENTRATION METHODS

Qualitative concentration techniques will be of greatest value in routine clinical diagnosis. They will detect most alimentary canal parasitisms and some of those from the respiratory tract. They may also aid in diagnosing certain skin manges of the dog, fox, and cat (see Figs. 1.42, 3.27).

The modified Sheather's method is reasonably rapid and is of value in the field of small animal practice and for the detection of certain parasitisms of horses, cattle, sheep, goats, swine, and poultry. Animal owners are usually interested in seeing parasitic forms under the microscope. Animal surgery is made safer by postponing operations on parasitized patients until such hosts are deparasitized. Veterinary hospital contamination and the transfer of many parasite species from patient to patient may be avoided through the isolation and treatment of those animals whose feces show evidence of a parasite burden.

A parasitized animal not exhibiting clinical symptoms may enter a veterinary hospital. Should parasitism develop to the clinical stage after that patient returns home, the owner may un-justly conclude that the animal acquired the parasites while in the hospital. Routine examination for parasites of all hospitalized pa-tients would avoid such criticism.

Fecal examination methods can and should be conducted in such a manner as to avoid contamination of the laboratory. To prevent the dissemination of odors, the samples should be kept covered as much as possible. Various commercial products are available for masking or neutralizing odors.

Concentration of parasite eggs or oocysts from feces may be accomplished in a number of ways. All methods depend on mixing the fecal sample with a liquid whose specific gravity is greater than that of most such forms but less than that of most of the fecal debris. Thus the parasite forms rise to the top of the flotation fluid by gravity — a process that may be hastened by centrifugation.

Flotation fluids may be of various composition. Those most commonly recommended include heavy solutions of sodium chloride, sucrose (cane or beet sugar), glycerine, zinc sulfate, zinc acetate, sodium nitrate, sodium acetate, or magnesium sulfate. None of these solutions is ideal for this purpose. Glycerine has too high a viscosity, hence flotation is slow. The saline solutions are low in viscosity but tend to dehydrate and thus distort parasite forms; also they crystallize rather quickly on the microslide. Solutions of high specific gravity (sp gr 1.400) will float too much debris, defeating the purpose for which they are intended.

Modified Sheather's Sugar Flotation Technique

Sheather (1923a) first proposed heavy sugar (sucrose) solution for fecal flotation technique. Our experience has shown that sugar solution (sp gr 1.200-1.300) is the most satisfactory flotation fluid available for routine qualitative clinical fecal examinations employing centrifugation. This solution will fail to float many of the eggs of tapeworms, flukes, and thorny-headed worms. This is not a serious objection because (1) tapeworm eggs usually leave the host enclosed within the worm's proglottides which may be seen grossly on or in the feces, and (2) except in certain localities, flukes and thorny-headed worms are not highly important parasites of domesticated animals. A technique for finding fluke eggs in feces is described on page 20.

Neither corn syrup nor dextrose solutions are suitable substitutes for granulated cane or beet sugar in fecal flotation techniques.

Materials

1. Centrifuge
2. Coverglasses
3. Coverglass forceps
4. Flotation solution
5. Glass-marking pencil
6. Headed glass rods or wire loop
7. Lens paper and xylene
8. Microscope
9. Microscope lamp

10. Microslides
11. Paper cups
12. Strainer
13. Test tubes
14. Test tube brush
15. Tongue depressors
16. Towels
17. Waste container
18. Water supply tube
19. Wooden apparatus block

1. <u>Centrifuge</u>. This may hold two or four or more tubes. Angle-type centrifuges are *not suitable* for fecal examination techniques. The tube holders should be large enough to accommodate test tubes of 10 ml capacity as well as the conventional conical centrifuge tubes of 15 ml capacity. The centrifuge should have a speed-regulating switch so that approximately 1500 revolutions per minute (rpm) may be maintained. The motor should be suitable to the electric current that is available (usually 115 volts alternating current). An electric timer-switch may be attached in the centrifuge line to break the current automatically at the end of the centrifuging period. A centrifuge suitable for conducting fecal examinations may also be used for other clinical laboratory procedures such as the preparation of blood and urine samples (see Fig. 1.8).

2. <u>Coverglasses.</u> Any 18 or 22 mm (¾ or ⅞ in) square glass or plastic coverglasses are suitable. The plastic covers are more economical. For best results in identifying microparasites, coverglasses must be used. Coverglasses may be dispensed from the wooden apparatus block.

3. <u>Coverglass forceps</u>. This should always be used when applying a coverglass to a specimen on a microslide (see Fig. 1.13).

4. <u>Flotation solution.</u>

    Granulated sugar (sucrose) . . . . 454 g (1 lb avdp)
    Tap water . . . . 355 ml (12 fl oz)
    40% formaldehyde solution, U.S.P. . . . . 6 ml

    Place the water in the upper half of a double boiler. Dissolve the sugar by stirring. The water in the lower half of the double boiler should be close to boiling. *Do not dissolve the sugar by means of direct heat*. Cool the sugar solution to room temperature. Then add the formaldehyde solution while stir-ring. The formaldehyde solution (or 1% liquefied phenol) acts as a deterrent to the growth of molds and yeasts. Store the sugar solution in stoppered bottles. It may be dispensed from a glass bottle or from an 8 oz plastic container such as that used for honey, catsup, or mustard.

5. Glass-marking pencil. This is for the identification of paper cups, test tubes, and microslides when more than one fecal sample is to be examined. Felt tip markers are suitable, provided the ink is not water soluble.

6. Headed glass rods. Various methods may be used for transferring parasites from the top of the centrifuged sample to a microslide. A circular wire loop about 10 mm in diameter has been recommended, but the results have not been satisfactory. The headed glass rod (Fig. 1.4) is made from a 15 cm (6 in) length of solid glass approximately 5 mm (³/₁₆ in) in diameter. In making the headed portion, one end of the rod is heated to redness in the flame of a Bunsen burner. The heated end is then quickly pressed against a warm, flat metal surface (such as the head of a hammer) until the rod end spreads to a diameter of about 10 mm (³/₈ in). The headed end should almost fill the open end of the test tube. After the rod has lost

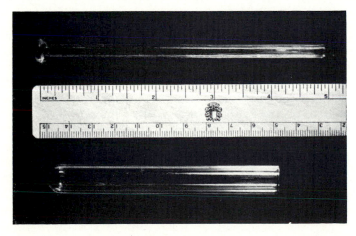

FIG. 1.4. Test tube *(below)* and headed glass rod *(above)* shown for comparative size.

its softness by cooling, the end is smoothed by again rotating it in the flame.

7. <u>Lens paper and xylene.</u> The oculars, objectives, condenser, and mirror of the microscope must be kept free from dust and other foreign matter. Only lens paper should be used for this purpose — either dry or, if necessary, dampened by water or by the solvent xylene. Lens paper squares of about 8 cm (3 in) may be dispensed from a covered glass or metal container. Used lens paper should always be discarded.

8. <u>Microscope.</u> Magnifications of 80–100 low power and 344–430 high power are most suitable for fecal examination. Therefore the microscope should be equipped with achromatic objectives of ×10 (16 mm) and ×43 (4 mm). The ocular (or oculars of binocular microscopes) should be of Huyghenian or widefield types of ×8 or ×10 magnification. A substage condenser of 1.25 numerical aperture is appropriate equipment. A mechanical stage and binocular body tube with matched oculars are not essential but will save the examiner's time and help to reduce eyestrain. The addition of an oil immersion objective will equip the microscope for all important clinical procedures, including hematology, bacteriology, and urology.

9. <u>Microscope lamp.</u> There are many types of microscope illuminators, including built-in illuminators of varying degrees of complexity. Any of these will be suitable for fecal examination. If the microscope is equipped with only a substage mirror, a simple illuminator will be suitable. For most pleasing results the microscope should be equipped with a blue filter in the substage light path or a blue bulb in the illuminator. Daylight or other diffuse light sources should not be relied on. The diagnostician is cautioned to select a sufficiently small aperture with the condenser diaphragm to avoid excessive light glare and consequent invisibility of eggs, many of which are quite transparent in light of high intensity; this is also true of cysts.

10. <u>Microslides.</u> Standard 75 x 25 mm (3 x 1 in) glass slides are used. They should be washed and dried before using (if not purchased clean) and may be reused repeatedly.

11. Paper cups. Disposable paper cups save time and prevent contamination. Cups of 90 ml (3 oz) capacity with nonfluted bottoms are recommended. They are available at most grocery stores. More durable cups are made from glass, plastic, aluminum, or stainless steel. These are usually available in 250 ml (8 oz) capacity. They should be cleaned with hot water and a brush before reuse.

12. Strainer. A small household tea strainer of metal wire may be used. It should have a mesh of about 12 per cm (30 per in), and the strainer should have an opening about 65 mm in diameter (see Fig. 1.7).

13. Test tubes. Those recommended are 10 cm (4 in) long by 12 mm (½ in) outside diameter, with a capacity of 10 ml (Fig. 1.4).

14. Test tube brush. The brush should be about 8 cm (3 in) long by 12 mm (½ in) in diameter. The bristles should be stiff.

15. Tongue depressors. These are standard items of wood supplied to the medical professions. They measure 15 cm long x 2 cm wide x 2 mm thick (6 in x ¾ in x ¹⁄₁₆ in). They are dispensed from a covered glass jar and are disposable.

16. Towels. Soft, woven towels, paper towels, or cellulose wipes are used for drying washed slides, tubes, and headed glass rods.

17. Waste container. Any convenient waterproof jar or pail may be used for the temporary disposal of fecal samples, paper cups, tongue depressors, and debris from the strainer. It is advisable to immerse these wastes in a disinfecting solution such as a quaternary ammonium compound.

18. Water supply tube. This is a test tube containing tap water and a medicine dropper.

19. Wooden apparatus block. This may be made by boring holes in a piece of wood (Fig. 1.5). After the holes are bored, the block is smoothed and coated with varnish or liquid plastic.

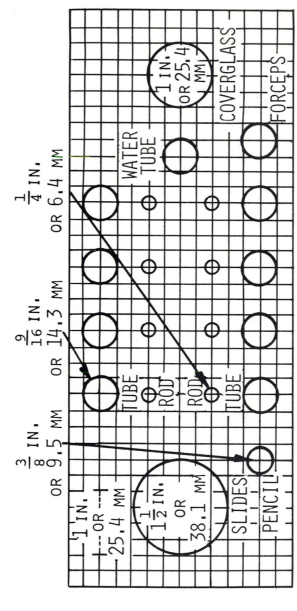

FIG. 1.5.   Wooden apparatus block, top view. Dimensions are: 9 in long, 3½ in wide, 1¾ in high (23 cm x 9 cm x 4.5 cm). The block accommodates 8 test tubes, 8 headed rods, microslides, coverglasses, water tube, coverglass forceps, and pencil. Crosslines are 4 to the inch.

Procedure

1. The fecal sample should be moist. If it is not, add enough water to soften it.

2. Place two paper cups on the table. Number them with the glass-marking pencil or otherwise identify them with the source of the sample.

3. Using a tongue depressor, transfer 1–2 g of feces to a paper cup (Fig. 1.6).

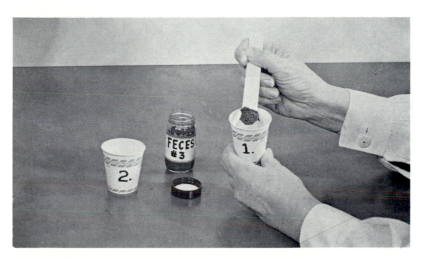

FIG. 1.6.   Using a tongue depressor, transfer 1–2 g of feces to a paper cup.

4. Add 15 ml of sugar solution, using a test tube for measuring volume (1½ tubefuls).

5. Using a tongue depressor, stir gently until the feces are thoroughly suspended in the sugar solution. Excess vigor in stirring will cause incorporation of air bubbles, making later observation of eggs and cysts difficult.

6. Pour the contents of the cup through the strainer into the second cup. Use the tongue depressor to stir and to gently press excess fluid from the debris remaining in the strainer (Fig. 1.7). Discard the debris into the waste container (not into a

sink) and clean the strainer *at once* in running water, preferably hot.

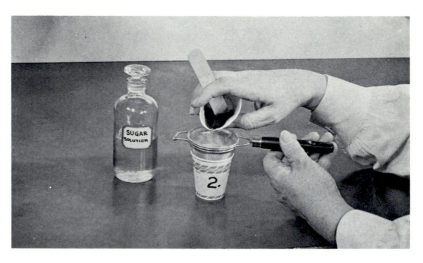

FIG. 1.7.   After adding and stirring in 15 ml of sugar solution, pour contents of the cup through a strainer into a second cup.

7. Using the glass-marking pencil, identify a test tube with the source of the sample.

8. Gently squeeze the rim of the paper cup to form a pouring spout. Gently agitate the strained feces by oscillating the cup. Immediately pour the mixture into the labeled test tube, filling it almost to the top (Fig. 1.8). If the strained sample is not agitated before transfer to the test tube, parasitic forms may be left in the bottom of the paper cup.

9. Place the test tube in the centrifuge. If necessary, add a balancing tube containing water. Gradually bring the speed of the centrifuge up to approximately 1500 rpm and maintain that speed for 3 minutes. A spring-actuated timer or an electric timer or timer switch are useful accessories for this step in the procedure.

      [If a centrifuge is not available, gravity flotation may be accomplished by allowing the test tube to remain undisturbed in the wooden apparatus block for several hours. The tube should be capped with a piece of aluminum foil to prevent evaporation and contamination.]

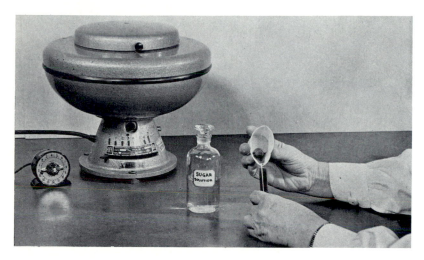

FIG. 1.8. Gently agitate the strained feces and immediately pour into a test tube, filling the tube almost to the top. Centrifuge the tube at 1500 rpm for 3 minutes.

10. While the centrifuge is in operation, place a clean microslide on the table. Center a drop of water on the microslide from a medicine dropper (Fig. 1.9). Wash and dry a headed glass rod.

11. Transfer the test tube from the centrifuge by holding the tube at the top. This avoids agitation of the contents. Gently place the test tube in the wooden apparatus block (Fig. 1.10). If after centrifugation there is a fatty layer or an excess of mineral particles on the top, a dry spud will pick this up and render the sample unfit for examination. In order to avoid having to discard the sample, first dip the spud into the drop of water on the slide. The eggs will adhere to the moist surface of the spud, leaving the excess debris in the tube.

12. Transfer a drop of sample from the test tube to the drop of water on the microslide (Fig. 1.11). To do this properly, hold the headed glass rod vertically over the tube, resting the elbow

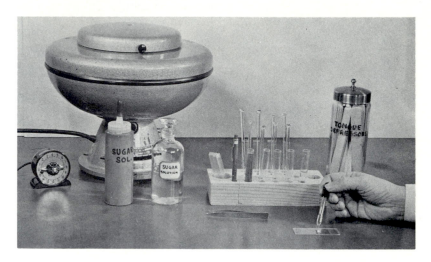

FIG. 1.9.   Place a drop of water in the center of a microslide.

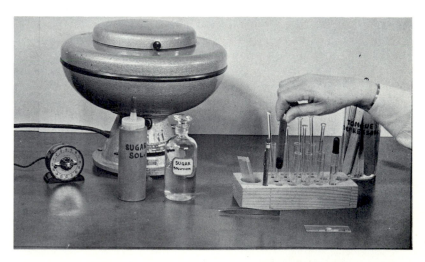

FIG. 1.10.   Remove the tube from the centrifuge and gently place it in the wooden apparatus block, holding it by the top.

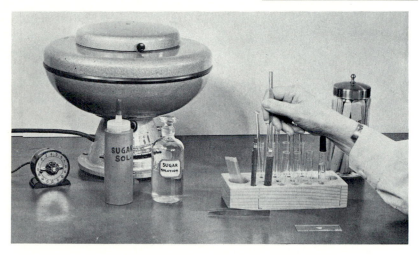

FIG. 1.11. Using a headed glass rod, remove a drop from the surface of the specimen in the tube. Quickly withdraw the rod after it has made full contact with the fluid.

on the table. Slowly lower the head of the glass rod onto the surface of the sample; then quickly withdraw the rod without making contact with the inside of the tube. This operation may require some practice. Hold the glass rod at about a 45-degree angle and rotate the headed end in the drop of water on the microslide; avoid contact of the spud and the slide (Fig. 1.12), thus washing off any parasite eggs or oocysts adhering to the rod. Replace the rod in the wooden apparatus block. It should be rinsed and dried before further use.

13. Pick up a coverglass by means of the coverglass forceps. Lower one edge of the coverglass onto the slide near the drop of suspension; then release the forceps as the coverglass is gently lowered onto the drop. The fluid should spread out evenly under the coverglass (Fig. 1.13). Too rapid an application of the coverglass will probably result in the formation of air bubbles, which may interfere with the microscopic examination of the specimen. *Avoid pressure on the coverglass, because parasitic forms are easily mutilated.*

14. Place the slide on the stage of the microscope so that the near right-hand corner of the coverglass is centered under the low-

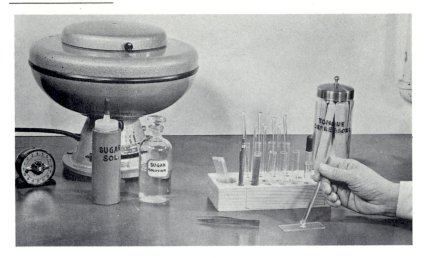

FIG. 1.12.   Wash the material from the head of the rod into the drop of water on the microslide. Rotate the rod in the water.

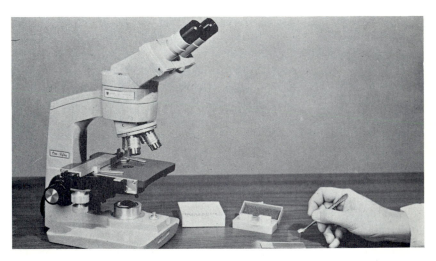

FIG. 1.13.   Using a coverglass forceps, place one edge of a coverglass into the fluid. Gently lower the coverglass onto the microslide. Do not press on the coverglass after it is in place.

magnification ($\times$10) objective. Focus on this corner. Adjust the substage condenser and diaphragm of the microscope so as to see a distinct image of the suspension under the coverglass. Using the low magnification ($\times$100), systematically move the microslide back and forth until the entire area of the coverglass has been scanned (Fig. 1.14). Objects having a resemblance to parasite forms may be centered and examined under high magnification ($\times$400). Always return to low magnification ($\times$100) for further scanning of the specimen.

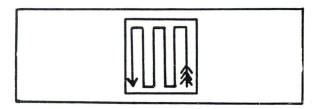

FIG. 1.14.   The material under the coverglass should be systematically examined, at $\times$ 100, according to diagram.

If worm eggs and coccidial oocysts or other protozoa are present in the same specimen, the coccidia and giardia, being smaller, tend to float upward until they rest directly beneath the coverglass. Therefore, when the worm eggs are in focus under high magnification ($\times$400), the coccidia and giardia, may be out of focus, and vice versa. All three types of parasitic forms may be brought clearly into focus by turning the fine-adjustment knob of the microscope.

Most of the photographs in Section 1 were taken at uniform magnifications of 100 and 410. A microscope usually used for clinical laboratory diagnosis has an apparent high-dry magnification field diameter of 18 cm (7 in). The high-magnification photographs are 9 cm (3½ in) in width. Therefore, each is about one-half the width of one apparent field of the microscope. This information may be useful in comparing the size of what is seen in the microscope at $\times$410 with that seen in the photographs.

Commercial Flotation System

In recent years a commercial outfit, Fecalyzer (Fig. 1.15) has been placed on the market. This is a complete system for collecting and examining fecal specimens for evidence of parasitism, based on the use of a sodium nitrate flotation medium. In the examination of feces of small animals, the results obtained are comparable to those of the modified Sheather's technique. However, for use with large animal feces, initial processing of the sample is necessary to remove fibrous debris. This procedure would seem to be most suitable for use in situations where each patient or client is assessed the cost of the kit used. (Information may be obtained from Evsco Pharmaceutical Corp., Oceanside, NY 11572.)

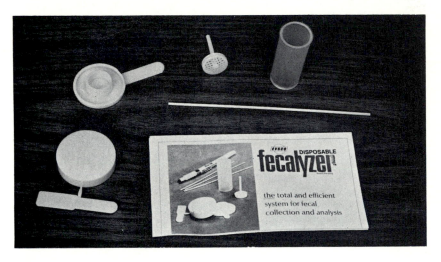

FIG. 1.15.   Fecalyzer components.

Modified Fluke Egg Technique

Since the early work of Cobb (1904), attempts have been made to find a simple, rapid method for demonstrating fluke eggs in the feces of domesticated animals. Several investigators have tried various types of flotation techniques but with inconsistent results because of the collapsibility of fluke eggs in solutions of high specific gravity. However, a modification of Sheather's sugar flotation technique has been used to demonstrate canine lung fluke *(Paragonimus kellicotti)* eggs in fecal samples. There was little or no collapse of the eggs.

The technique of Dennis, Stone, and Swanson (1954) appears to be relatively simple for the *quantitative* demonstration of fluke eggs. It requires about one-half hour to perform. The following modification of this method is useful for *qualitative* clinical diagnosis.

Materials

1. Centrifuge tubes
2. Centrifuge tube and test tube block
3. Coverglasses
4. Detergent solution
5. Fecal containers
6. Filter pump
7. Funnel-strainer
8. Microscope
9. Microslides
10. Pipette
11. Stirring rod
12. Test tubes
13. Tincture of iodine
14. Tongue depressors
15. Wash bottle

1. Centrifuge tubes. Each tube has a capacity of 50 ml (1.7 oz). It is made of plain glass and has a rounded bottom and a pourout lip. The diameter is 28.5 mm (1⅛ in) and the length is 12 cm (4¾ in).

2. Centrifuge tube and test tube block. This is a piece of wood approximately 6 cm (2⅜ in) thick with holes bored 3 cm (1⅛ in) in diameter for the centrifuge tubes and 2 cm (¾ in) for the test tubes (one hole of each size is needed for one sample).

3. Coverglasses. These are standard 22 mm (⅞ in) squares of plastic or glass.

4. Detergent solution.
   Liquid household detergent .... 5 ml
   Tap water .... 995 ml (33.6 fl oz)
   1% solution alum (aluminum potassium
      sulfate, U.S.P.) .... 8 drops

5. Fecal containers. These are wide-mouthed, screw-capped or stoppered glass jars of at least 60 ml (2 oz) capacity.

6. Filter pump. This uses water faucet pressure to produce suction (Richards filter pump). A decanting bottle using mouth suction or a bulb syringe of about 30 ml (1 oz) capacity may be used in place of the filter pump.

7. Funnel-strainer. This is a tin- or zinc-coated funnel 9 cm (3½ in) in diameter, with an 80-mesh disk of copper screen soldered 25 mm (1 in) from the top.

8. Microscope. A clinical microscope and lamp are suitable.

9. Microslides. These are standard 75 x 25 mm (3 x 1 in) glass slides.

10. Pipette. This has a capacity of 2 ml.

11. Stirring rod. This may be of wood, glass, or metal. Standard disposable wooden applicator sticks may be used. The stirring rod should be 15 cm (6 in) long, with a diameter of about 2 mm (³⁄₃₂ in).

12. Test tubes. These are stout-walled glass tubes of 30 ml (1 oz) capacity. They measure 150 x 18 mm (6 x ¾ in).

13. Tincture of iodine, U.S.P. This is dispensed from a medicine dropper.

14. Tongue depressors. These are the standard 15 cm (6 in) length.

15. Wash bottle. This is a standard laboratory item of 1 liter (32 oz) capacity.

Procedure

1. Using a tongue depressor, mix the fecal sample thoroughly; if it is very dry, add cold tap water to form a pasty mass.

2. Place about 1 g of the mixed feces in a 30 ml (1 oz) test tube.

3. Add 15 ml (½ oz) detergent solution. Mix well with a stirring rod. To avoid sudsing, do not shake.

4. Strain the mixture through the funnel-strainer into a 50 ml (1.7 oz) centrifuge tube.

5. Rinse the test tube with more detergent solution and strain.

6. Pour enough detergent solution in a flooding, swirling motion through the feces in the funnel-strainer to fill the centrifuge tube.

7. Allow the tubed mixture to stand for 5-15 minutes.

8. Decant three-fourths of the liquid portion from the centrifuge tube.

9. Rewash the fecal material in the funnel-strainer to refill the centrifuge tube, in order to obtain any eggs trapped previously. Discard the funnel contents.

10. Again allow the tubed mixture to stand for 5–15 minutes.

11. Again decant all liquid down to about 2–3 ml. Do not disturb the sediment.

12. Add 1–3 drops tincture of iodine to the sediment, allowing the tube to stand for 2–5 minutes.

13. Using a pipette, transfer the sediment to one or more microslides and apply coverglasses.
(Note: Dennis et al. [1954] recommend placing all of the sediment in a standard petri dish, adding tap water to make 15–20 ml, and searching for eggs with a binocular dissecting microscope magnifying × 18 or higher.)

14. Search the sediment on the slide or slides, using a clinical microscope magnifying × 100.

QUANTITIVE METHODS
     Various techniques have been proposed for the determination of the *number* of parasite eggs or coccidial oocysts per gram of feces. Such methods are of value in the study of parasite life cycles or in determining the effects of experimental therapy for the removal of gastrointestinal parasites. Quantitative fecal techniques are of little value in clinical diagnosis; therefore, such methods are not included in this publication.

(References for Section 1 will be found on pages 239–50.)

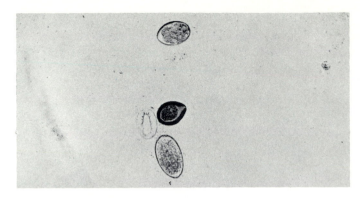

FIG. 1.16. Oocyst of *Eimeria leuckarti*, two strongyle eggs, and an egg of *Strongyloides westeri*. ×100. Oocyst size 74.1 x 48.7–54.6 μm.

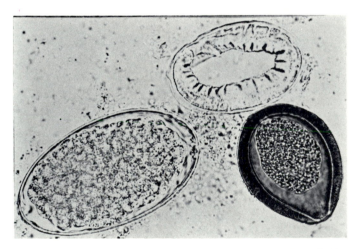

FIG. 1.17. Oocyst of *Eimeria leuckarti*, a *Strongyloides westeri* egg, and a strongyle egg. ×410. The oocyst is dark brown.

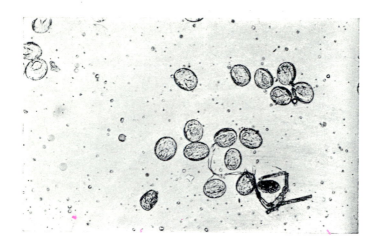

FIG. 1.18.   Eggs of *Paranoplocephala mamillana,* the small tapeworm of equines. Eggs of the other tapeworms of equines *(Anoplocephala magna* and *Anoplocephala perfoliata)* are similar to these. ×100. Egg size 50–60 μm.

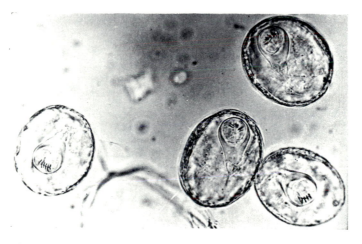

FIG. 1.19.   Eggs of *Paranoplocephala mamillana*. The eggs enclose a pear-shaped embryo having six hooklets. ×410.

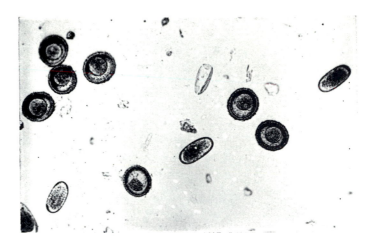

FIG. 1.20.   Eggs of *Parascaris equorum,* the ascarid of equines. The eggshells are rough and thick and yellow to brown in color. Also included are three strongyle eggs. ×100. Egg size 90–100 μm.

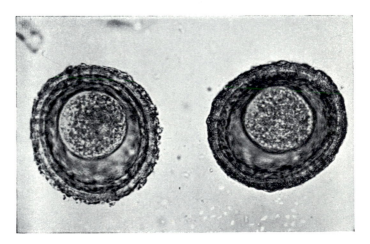

FIG. 1.21.   Eggs of *Parascaris equorum.* Ascarid eggs may be found lacking the external shell covering, hence they appear colorless. ×410.

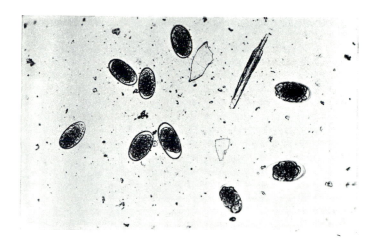

FIG. 1.22. Eggs from several species of strongyles of equines. Thirty-nine species of these nematodes have been reported from the large intestine of horses, asses, and mules in North America. The eggs of all species are similar. ×100. Egg size 70–85 x 40–47 μm.

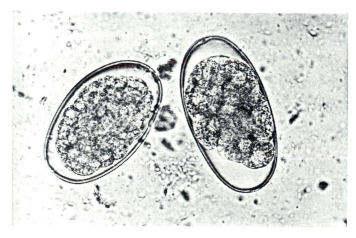

FIG. 1.23. Eggs from two species of strongyles of equines. ×410.

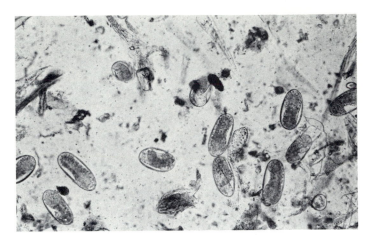

FIG. 1.24. Equine strongyle eggs 12 hours after passage from the host. The cells are now too numerous to be recognized individually. ×100.

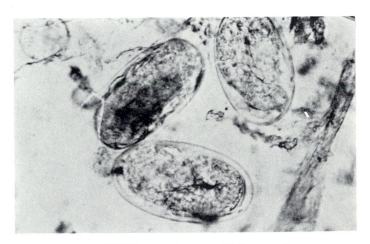

FIG. 1.25. Equine strongyle eggs 12 hours after passage from the host. ×400. This appearance indicates the sample was not fresh. Contamination by free-living nematodes may occur as a source of confusion if such samples are recovered from the ground.

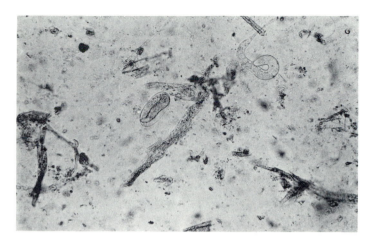

FIG. 1.26. Equine strongyle eggs 36 hours after passage from the host. Development has already progressed to vermiform larval stage. ×100.

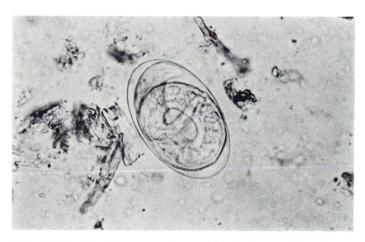

FIG. 1.27. Equine strongyle egg after 36 hours of development. ×400. Such development indicates that the fecal sample was not fresh. Misdiagnosis may arise since some helminths pass eggs already in this stage. Gastrointestinal nematodes of cattle behave in a similar manner.

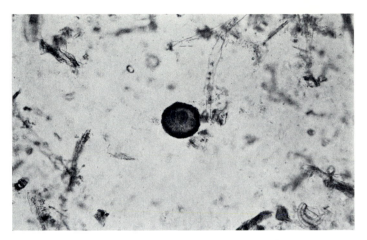

FIG. 1.28.   Egg of *Parascaris equorum*, the large round-worm of horses. This egg is in the eight-cell stage 24 hours after passage from the host. Many ascarids develop rapidly in the early stages. × 100.

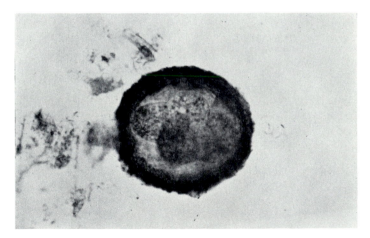

FIG. 1.29.   Egg of *Parascaris equorum*. The eight-cell stage is noticeable 24 hours after passage. × 400.

FIG. 1.30.   Eggs of *Draschia megastoma,* one of the three larger gastric nematodes of horses. These eggs are from the exudate in a gastric abscess containing adult worms. Larvae are found in feces. ×100.

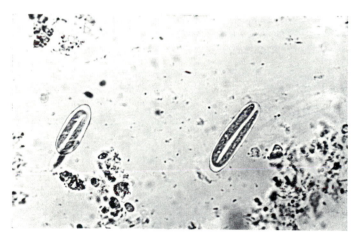

FIG. 1.31.   Eggs of *Draschia megastoma.* ×410.

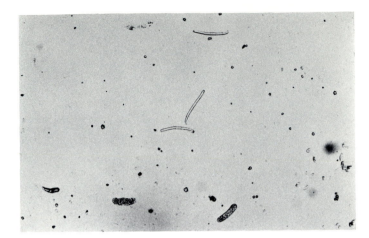

FIG. 1.32.　Eggs of *Habronema muscae*, one of the three larger gastric nematodes of horses. These eggs are elongated, embryonated when laid, and surrounded by a very thin membranous shell. ×100. Egg size 40-50 x 10-12 μm.

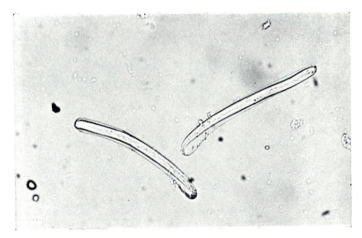

FIG. 1.33.　Eggs of *Habronema muscae*. ×410.

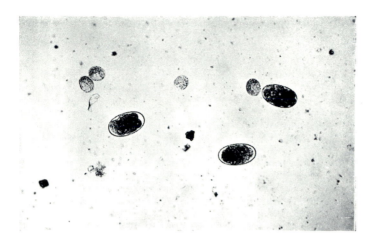

FIG. 1.34.   Eggs of *Strongyloides westeri,* the intestinal threadworm of horses. The three larger eggs are those of strongyles. ×100. Egg size 40–50 x 32–40 μm.

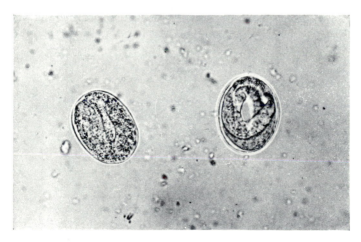

FIG. 1.35.   Eggs of *Strongyloides westeri.* These eggs are embryonated when laid. ×410.

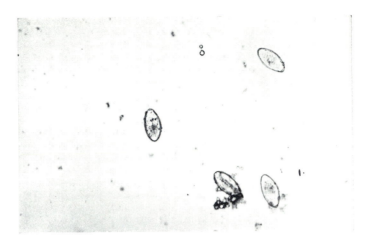

FIG. 1.36. Eggs of *Oxyuris equi,* the rectal worm of horses. These eggs may be found in the feces, but examination of anal scrapings is a more accurate method of diagnosis. ×100. Egg size 90 x 42 μm.

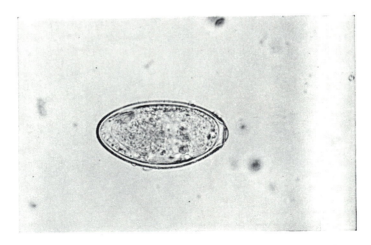

FIG. 1.37. Egg of *Oxyuris equi.* Note the operculum (cap) at one end. ×410.

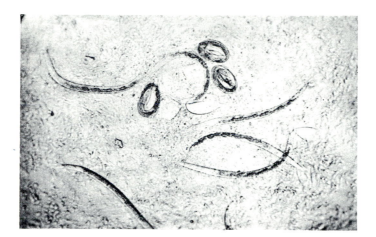

FIG. 1.38.   Eggs and larvae of *Dictyocaulus arnfieldi*, the lungworm of horses. These were taken from bronchial exudate. Only the larvae are found in the feces. ×100. Egg size 80–100 x 50–60μm.

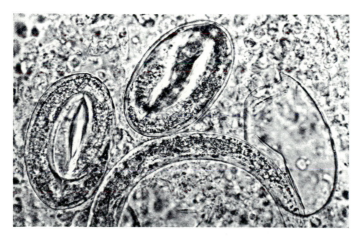

FIG. 1.39.   Eggs, part of a larva, and an empty eggshell of *Dictyocaulus arnfieldi.* ×410.

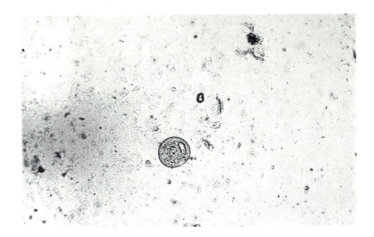

FIG. 1.40.   A cyst of *Buxtonella sulcata* of cattle. This is the resting stage of a large ciliated protozoon of the cecum of cattle. Nothing is known regarding its possible pathogenicity. It is commonly found in cattle feces. ×100. Trophozoites size 60–138 x 46–100 μm.

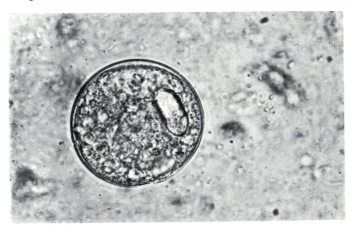

FIG. 1.41.   *Buxtonella sulcata* cyst. ×410.

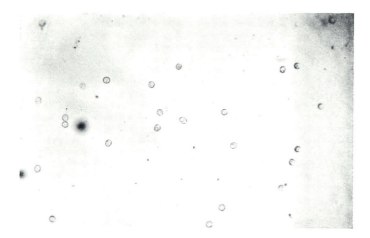

FIG. 1.42.   Oocysts of *Eimeria zuernii,* one of the more pathogenic of the eleven species of coccidia of cattle in North America. ×100. Oocyst size 15–22 x 13–18 μm.

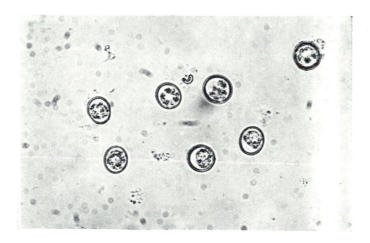

FIG. 1.43.   Oocysts of *Eimeria zuernii.* ×410.

FIG. 1.44.   Oocysts of *Eimeria auburnensis,* a coccidium of cattle. The color is yellowish brown. One smooth-walled and two rough-walled cysts are shown. ×100. Oocyst size 32–46 x 20–26μm.

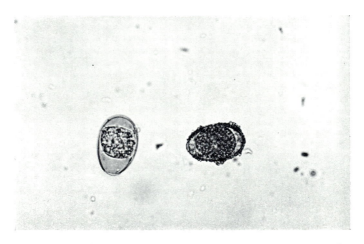

FIG. 1.45.   Oocysts of *Eimeria auburnensis.* Smooth-walled form at the left; rough-walled form at the right. ×410.

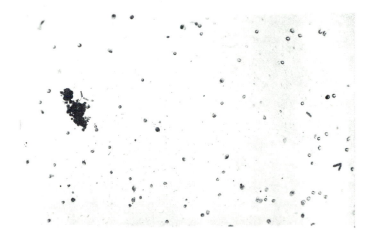

FIG. 1.46. *Giardia bovis,* a flagellate protozoon of cattle. These motile forms are taken from the contents of the small intestine. The forms found in feces are spherical nonmotile cysts. Similar giardias are found in sheep, goats, dogs, and cats. ×100. 9–21 μm long, 5–15 μm wide, 2–4 μm thick.

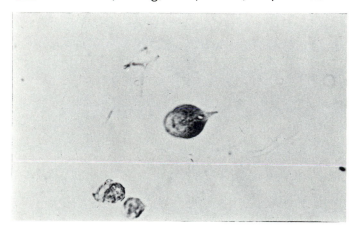

FIG. 1.47. *Giardia bovis* showing the two posterior flagella. ×410.

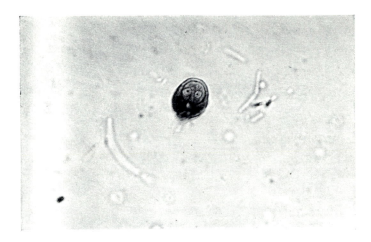

FIG. 1.48. *Giardia bovis* showing the ventral sucking disc and the two nuclei. ×410. 9–21 μm long, 5–15 μm wide, 2–4 μm thick.

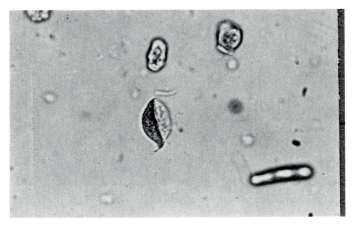

FIG. 1.49. *Giardia bovis,* oblique view to show the ventral concavity and posterior flagella. ×410.

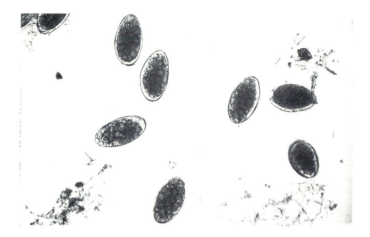

FIG. 1.50.   Eggs of *Fasciola hepatica,* the common liver fluke of sheep, goats, cattle, and swine; also of bison, deer, and rabbits. ×100. Egg size 130–150 x 63–90 μm.

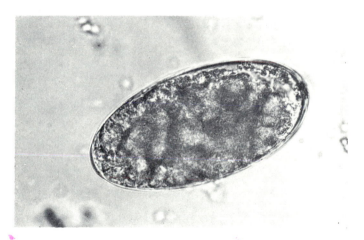

FIG. 1.51.   Egg of *Fasciola hepatica.* ×410.

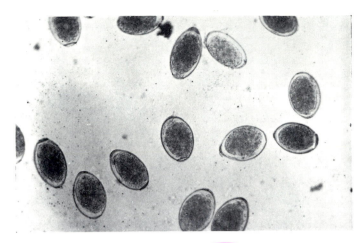

FIG. 1.52. Eggs of *Fascioloides magna,* the large American liver fluke of sheep, goats, cattle, and rarely of horses; also of bison, deer, elk, and moose. Because cattle are abnormal hosts, the eggs usually remain in the liver. ×100. Egg size 109–168 x 75–96 μm.

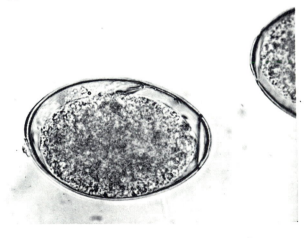

FIG. 1.53. Egg of *Fascioloides magna*. Note the operculum at one end. ×410.

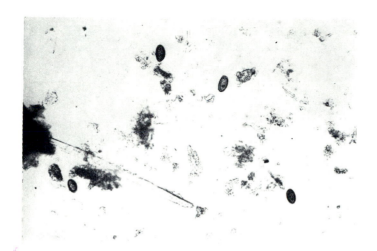

FIG. 1.54.   Eggs of *Dicrocoelium dendriticum*, the lancet liver fluke of cattle, sheep, deer, and woodchucks. ×100. Egg size 36–45 x 22–30 μm.

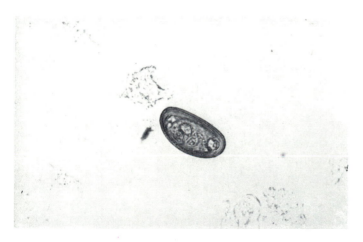

FIG. 1.55.   Egg of *Dicrocoelium dendriticum*. ×410.

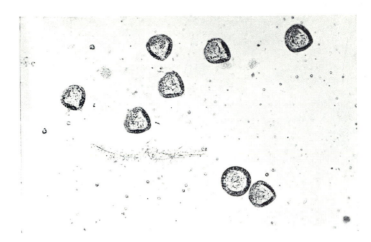

FIG. 1.56. Eggs of *Moniezia expansa,* one of the two species of large tapeworms of cattle, sheep, and goats; also of mountain sheep, moose, antelopes, and musk ox. The eggs of *Moniezia benedeni* are similar to these. ×100. Egg size 56–67 μm in diameter.

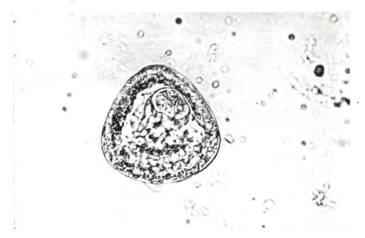

FIG. 1.57. Egg of *Moniezia expansa.* Note the pear-shaped embryo which contains six hooklets. ×410.

Because of the similarity in egg morphology of a number of the gastrointestinal nematodes of cattle, sheep, and goats in North America it is difficult to identify the worm by a fecal examination. The following table of egg measurements may be useful:

Bunostomum trigonocephalum	82–97 x 47–57 μm
Chabertia ovina	83–100 x 47–59 μm
Cooperia curticei	70–82 x 35–41 μm
Cooperia oncophora	83.2 x 39.7 μm average
Cooperia pectinata	70–80 x 36 μm
Cooperia punctata	76.6 x 32.2 μm average
Haemonchus contortus	70–85 x 41–48 μm
Oesophagostomum columbianum	73–89 x 34–45 μm
Ostertagia circumcincta	85–103 x 44–56 μm
Ostertagia ostertagi	80–85 x 40–45 μm
Trichostrongylus axei	79–92 x 31–41 μm
Trichostrongylus capricola	79–98 x 38–44 μm
Trichostrongylus colubriformis	79–101 x 39–47 μm
Trichostrongylus vitrinus	93–118 x 41–52 μm

Note: Cattle, sheep, and goats in North America harbor 27 species of gastrointestinal nematodes, the eggs of which are similar in morphology. These worms include the following: Haemonchus (2 species), Trichostrongylus (5 species), Cooperia (7 species), Oesophagostomum (3 species), Bunostomum (2 species), Ostertagia (6 species), Pseudostertagia (1 species), and Chabertia (1 species). Drawings of these eggs are found in a bulletin by Shorb (1939). Measurements of some of these eggs are found in the chart above.

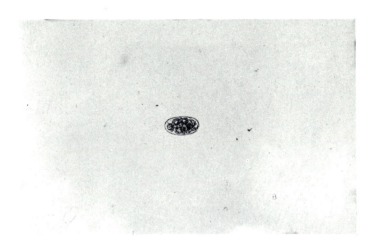

FIG. 1.58.   Egg of *Haemonchus contortus*, the common or "twisted" stomach worm of cattle, sheep, and goats. ×100. Egg size 70–85 x 41–48 µm.

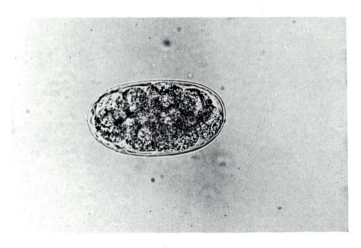

FIG. 1.59.   Egg of *Haemonchus contortus*. ×400.

FIG. 1.60. Egg of *Nematodirus spathiger*, a thread-necked nematode of the small intestine of cattle, sheep, and goats; also of bighorn sheep, and deer. ×100. Egg size 150–230 x 80–110 μm.

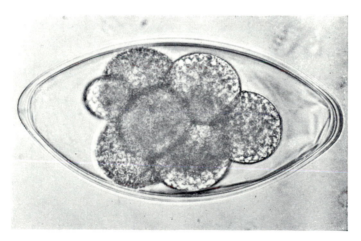

FIG. 1.61. Egg of *Nematodirus spathiger*. The embryonic mass is in the eight-celled stage. Note the thickened shell at the poles. ×400.

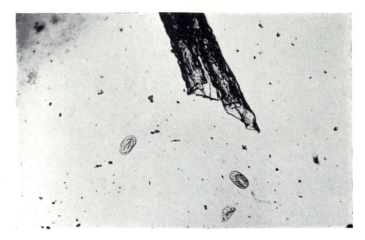

FIG. 1.62.   Eggs of *Strongyloides papillosus,* a thread-worm of the small intestine of cattle, sheep, goats, and rabbits. ×100. Egg size 40-60 x 20-25 μm.

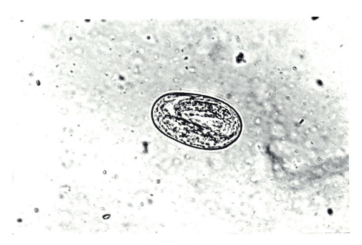

FIG. 1.63.   Egg of *Strongyloides papillosus.* The eggs of this nematode are embryonated when laid. ×410.

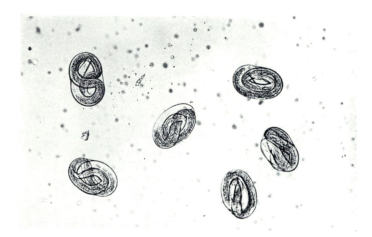

FIG. 1.64. Eggs of *Dictyocaulus filaria,* a lungworm of sheep, goats, and deer. These eggs were taken from bronchial exudate. They are embryonated when laid but usually hatch before they leave the host with the feces. ×100. Egg size 112–138 x 69–90 μm.

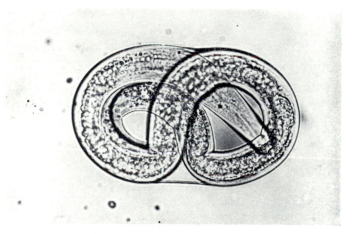

FIG. 1.65.   Egg of *Dictyocaulus filaria.* ×410.

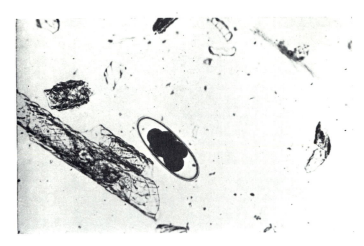

FIG. 1.66.   Egg of *Marshallagia marshalli*, a stomach worm of sheep and goats. ×100. Egg size 178–217 x 78–100 μm.

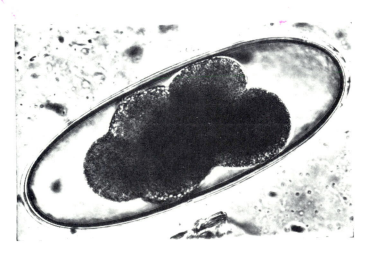

FIG. 1.67.   Egg of *Marshallagia marshalli*. ×410.

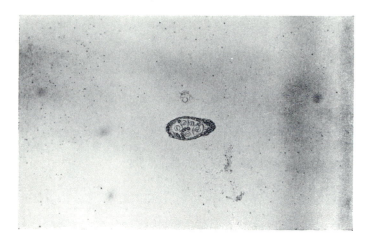

FIG. 1.68. A packet (parauterine) containing eggs of *Thysanosoma actinioides*, the fringed tapeworm of sheep and goats; also of antelope, deer, elk, moose. These egg packets usually leave the host within the tapeworm segments, hence are seldom found during routine fecal examination. ×100. Egg size 19.25–26.95 μm in diameter.

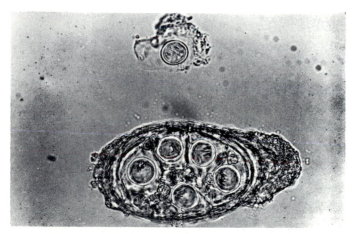

FIG. 1.69. A packet (parauterine) containing eggs of *Thysanosoma actinioides*. Five eggs are visible within the packet and one egg is free. ×410.

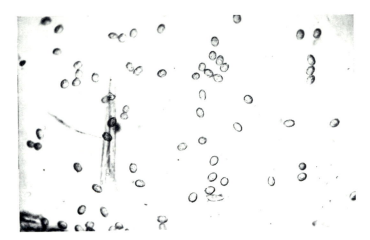

FIG. 1.70. Oocysts of *Eimeria ovina* (syn.: *E. arloingi*), one of the more pathogenic species of coccidia of sheep in North America. The color varies from pale yellow to yellowish green. ×100. Oocyst size 17–42 x 13–27 μm.

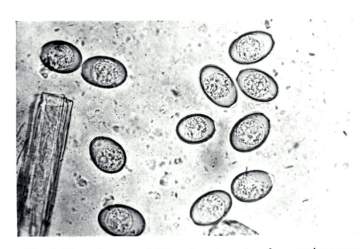

FIG. 1.71. Oocysts of *Eimeria ovina*. A polar cap is present at one end of the cyst. ×410.

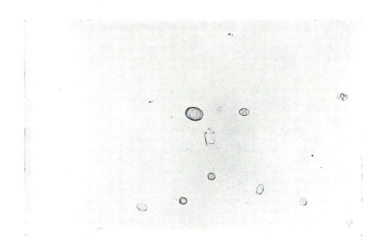

FIG. 1.72.   Oocysts of *Eimeria intricata* and *Eimeria ovina* (syn.: *E. arloingi*), coccidia of sheep and bighorn sheep. The large oocyst is that of *E. intricata,* the color of which is dark brown. ×100. Oocyst size 39–54 x 27–36 μm.

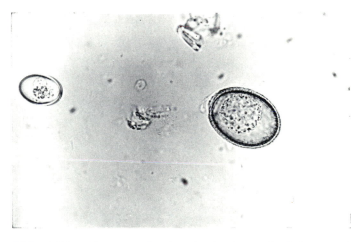

FIG. 1.73.   Oocysts of *Eimeria intricata (right)* and of *Eimeria ovina (left).* ×410.

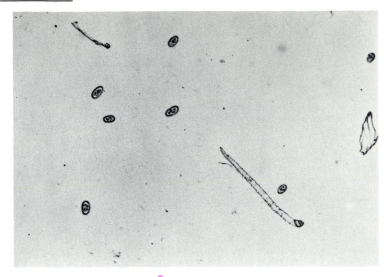

FIG. 1.74. **Pseudoparasite. Plant hair** from sheep feces.
These may be mistaken for larval nematodes. Others have a
smooth outer surface. × 100.

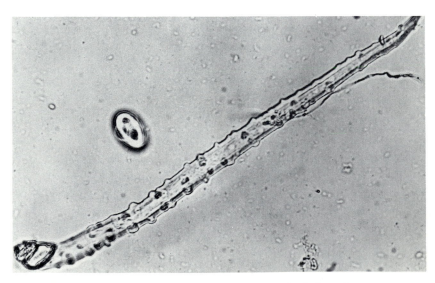

FIG. 1.75. Plant hair from sheep feces. Note the left end
of the hair where it is broken from the main stem. × 410.

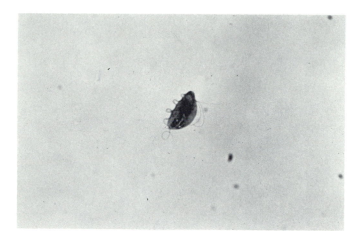

FIG. 1.76. *Trichomonas suis,* the swine nasal trichomonad. The appearance is also characteristic for species occurring in feces from most domestic animals. ×800.

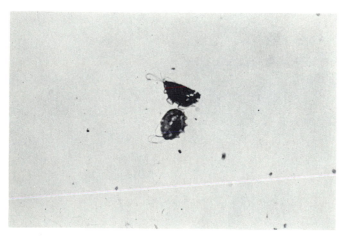

FIG. 1.77.   *Trichomonas suis.* ×800.

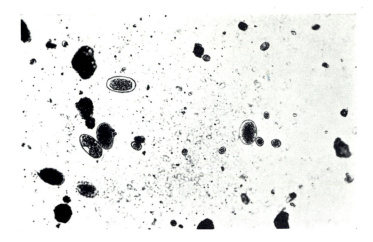

FIG. 1.78. Oocysts of *Eimeria* sp., coccidia of swine. Several species are shown. The eggs are those of *Oesophagostomum* sp., one of the nodule worms. ×100. *Eimeria debliecki* oocysts 13–29 x 13–19 μm.

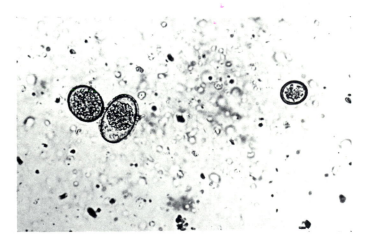

FIG. 1.79. Oocysts of *Eimeria* sp. Three species are shown. ×410.

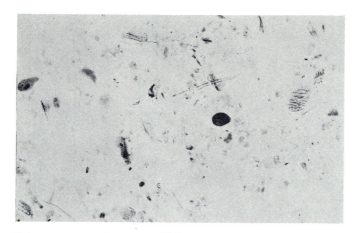

FIG. 1.80. *Balantidium coli,* a ciliated protozoon found in the cecum and colon of swine, causing balantidiosis. This is the mature form (trophozoite) which may be seen in the feces of swine having diarrhea. In normal swine this parasite appears in the feces as a spherical cyst about one-half the size of the mature form. This species may cause dysentery in man and monkeys. ×100. Trophozoite size 30–150 x 25–120 μm.

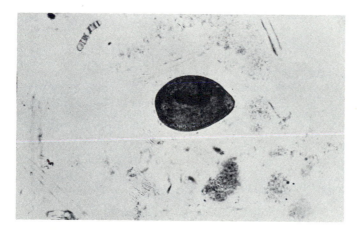

FIG. 1.81. *Balantidium coli* trophozoite (mature form). Iron hematoxylin stain. ×410.

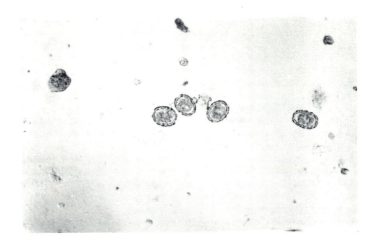

FIG. 1.82.   Eggs of *Ascaris suum*, the ascarid of swine. × 100. Egg size 50–75 x 40–50 μm.

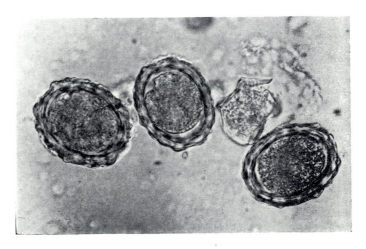

FIG. 1.83.   Eggs of *Ascaris suum*. × 400.

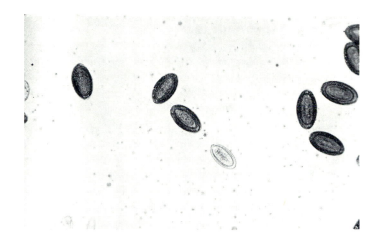

FIG. 1.84.   Eggs of *Macracanthorhynchus hirudinaceus,*
the thorny-headed worm of swine.   ×100. Egg size
67–100 x 40–65 μm.

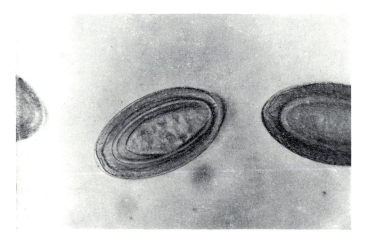

FIG. 1.85.   Eggs of *Macracanthorhynchus hirudinaceus.*
The embryo is surrounded by three shells. The outer shell is
dark brown. ×100.

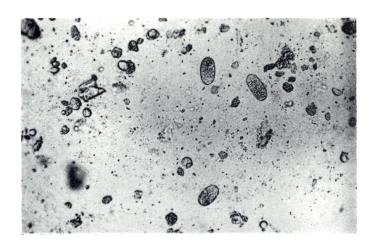

FIG. 1.86. Eggs of *Oesophagostomum* sp., one of four species of nodule worms of swine. ×100. Egg size 73–89 x 34–45 μm.

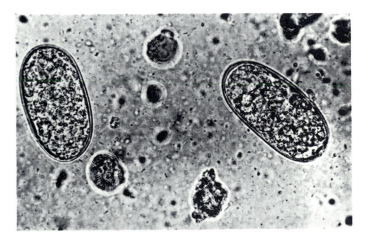

FIG. 1.87. Eggs of *Oesophagostomum* sp. ×410.

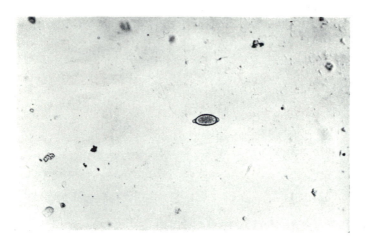

FIG. 1.88.   Egg of *Trichuris suis,* the whipworm of swine.
×100. Egg size 50–60 x 21–25 μm.

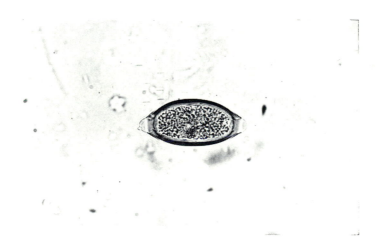

FIG. 1.89.   Egg of *Trichuris suis.* ×400.

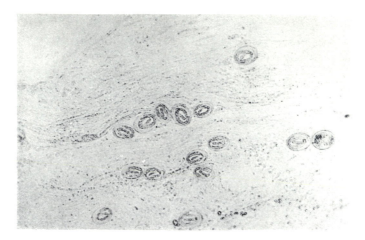

FIG. 1.90. Eggs of *Metastrongylus apri,* one of the lungworms of swine. These were removed from the bronchial exudate but may also be found in the feces. The eggs are embryonated when laid. ×100. Egg size 45–57 x 38–41 μm.

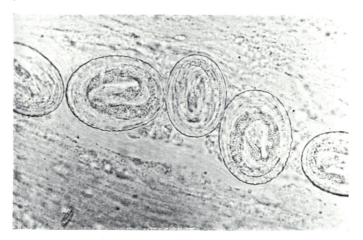

FIG. 1.91. Eggs of *Metastrongylus apri.* ×400.

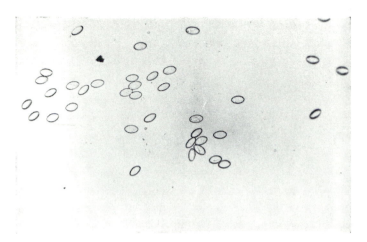

FIG. 1.92.   Eggs of *Ascarops strongylina,* one of the stomach worms of swine. ×100. Egg size 34–39 x 20 µm.

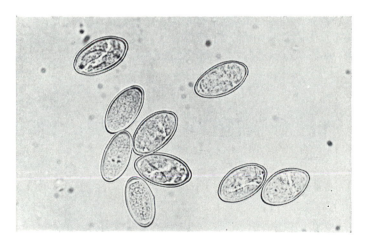

FIG. 1.93.   Eggs of *Ascarops strongylina.* ×410.

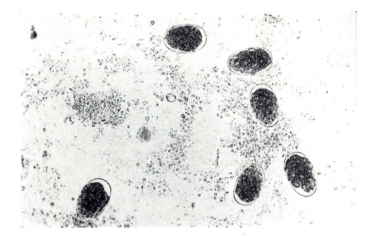

FIG. 1.94. Eggs of *Stephanurus dentatus*, the kidney worm of swine. These eggs are found in urinary sediment and occasionally in the feces. × 100. Egg size 100 x 60 μm.

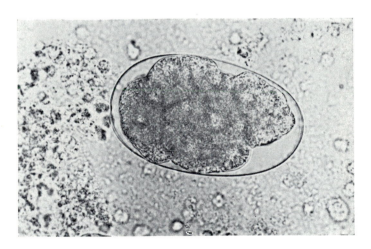

FIG. 1.95. Egg of *Stephanurus dentatus*. × 410.

FIG. 1.96. Oocysts of *Isospora* sp., one of the coccidia of dogs, cats, foxes, and minks. This coccidium is often referred to as the smaller form of *Isospora bigemina*. The oocysts are not sporulated when found in fresh feces. ×100. Small oocyst size 10–14 x 7–9 μm; large oocyst size 18–20 x 14–16 μm.

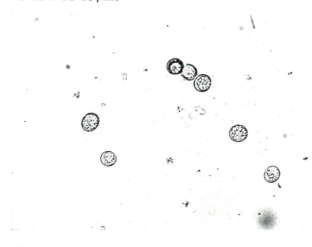

FIG. 1.97. Oocysts of *Isospora* sp. ×410.

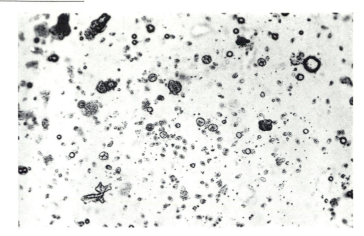

FIG. 1.98. Sporulated oocysts and sporocysts of *Isospora bigemina*, a coccidium of dogs, cats, and foxes. The larger oocysts are those of *Isospora ohioensis*. ×100. *Ohioensis* oocysts 20–25 x 15–20 μm.

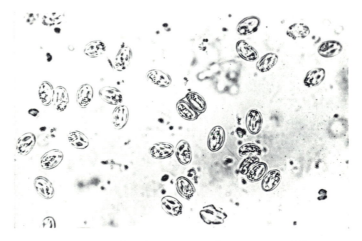

FIG. 1.99. Sporulated oocysts and sporocysts of *Isospora bigemina*. This coccidium is often referred to as the larger form of this species. The oocysts sporulate before leaving the body of the host; the delicate oocyst wall frequently ruptures, liberating the two sporocysts, each of which contains four sporozoites. ×410.

Note: Isospora rivolta of cats is identical to *Isospora ohioensis*, but each species is host specific. It appears that *Isospora bigemina* can no longer be regarded as a single species. At least three species, *Sarcocystis bigemina*, *Isospora heydorni*, and *Isospora wallacei* have been proposed for various forms of *I. bigemina* (see: Levine, 1977; Frenkel, 1977; Dubey, 1976). A new genus, *Cystoisospora*, has even been proposed in place of *Isospora* in dogs and cats. We are retaining the designation *Isospora bigemina*, and the genus *Isospora*, smaller form, until the taxonomy of these forms has been more clearly defined.

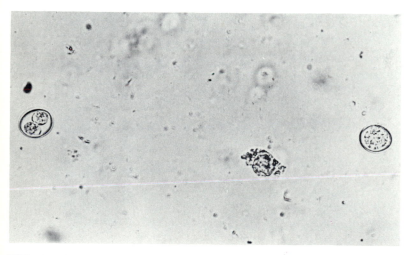

FIG. 1.100. Oocysts of *Isospora ohioensis,* one of the coccidia of dogs. These oocysts are intermediate in size between
those of *I. wallacei* and *I. felis.* ×100. Oocyst size
20–25 x 15–20 μm.

FIG. 1.101. Oocyst of *Isospora ohioensis.* ×410.

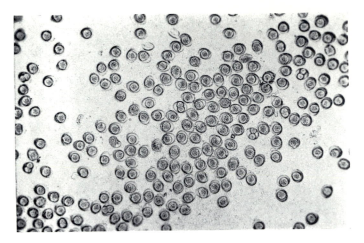

FIG. 1.102. Oocysts of *Isospora canis*, the largest species of the coccidia of dogs. ×100. Oocyst size 32–53 x 26–43 μm.

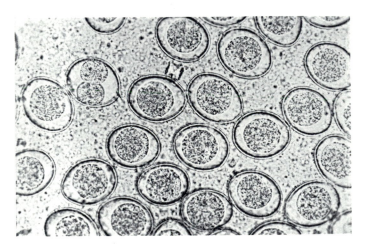

FIG. 1.103. Oocysts of *Isospora canis*. One shows beginning sporulation. ×410.

Note: Isospora felis of cats is identical to *Isospora canis*, but each species is host specific. A flagellate protozoon, *Giardia canis*, has been reported from the small intestine of dogs, and the same or a similar species, *Giardia felis*, from cats. Their morphology is similar to that of *Giardia bovis*, shown in Figs. 1.46–1.49.

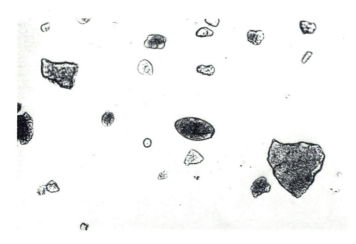

FIG. 1.104.   Egg of *Paragonimus kellicotti,* the lung fluke of dogs, cats, foxes, goats, swine, and rarely of man; also of bobcats, minks, muskrats, opossums, raccoons, and skunks. ×100. Egg size 75–118 x 42–67 μm.

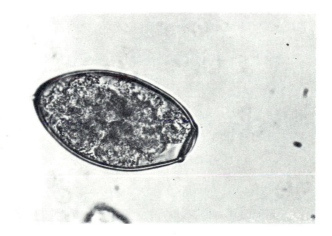

FIG. 1.105.   Egg of *Paragonimus kellicotti.* Note the prominent lid (operculum) at the right. ×410.

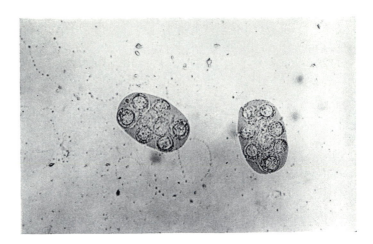

FIG. 1.106. Packets of *Dipylidium caninum* eggs, the double-pored tapeworm of dogs, cats, foxes, coyotes, and rarely of man. The smaller packets may be detected by flotation; the larger packets sink when the specimen is centrifuged. This is the only tapeworm of the dog, cat, and fox whose eggs are contained in packets. Each packet contains 1–63 eggs. ×100. Egg size 35 x 60 μm.

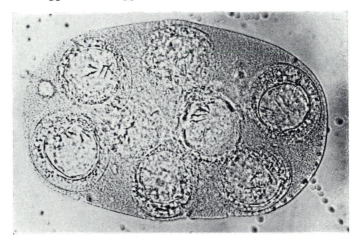

FIG. 1.107. A packet of eggs of *Dipylidium caninum*. Each egg in the packet is provided with six hooklets. ×400.

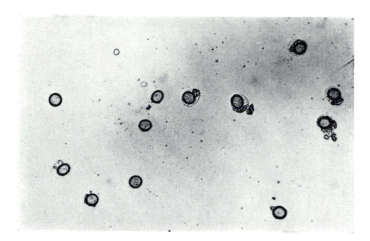

FIG. 1.108.   Eggs of *Taenia pisiformis*, one of the common rabbit cyst tapeworms of dogs, cats, and foxes; also of bobcats, coyotes, and wolves. In general, the eggs of tapeworms leave the host within the ripe tapeworm segments. However, eggs may be found during microscopic examination of feces. ×100. Egg size 37 x 32 μm.

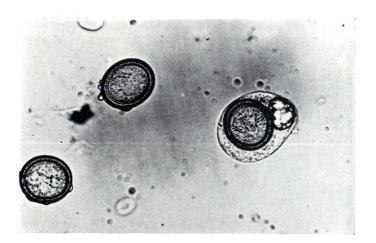

FIG. 1.109.   Eggs of *Taenia pisiformis*. Note the radially striated shell and the embryonic hooklets. The egg at the right is contained within an embryonic membrane. ×400.

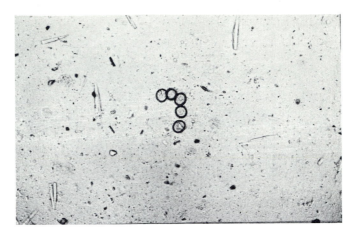

FIG. 1.110.   Five eggs of *Echinococcus granulosus*, the hydatid cyst tapeworm now rarely reported in dogs, foxes, and cats; also of coyotes, mountain lions, and wolves. Note the similarity of these eggs to those in Figs. 1.108, 1.109, 1.157, 1.158. ×100. Egg size 32-36 x 25-30 μm.

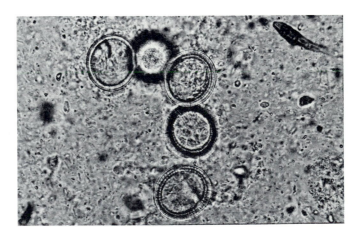

FIG. 1.111.   Eggs of *Echinococcus granulosus*. Three eggs are in focus; the other two are situated lower, hence are not distinct. ×410.

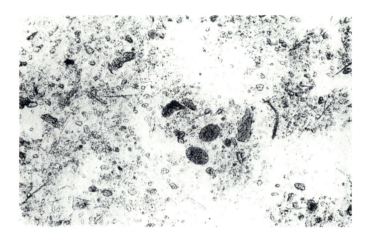

FIG. 1.112.   Eggs of *Dibothriocephalus latus*, the broad fish tapeworm of dogs, foxes, cats, and man; also of bears, minks, seals, sea lions, walruses, and wolves. ×100. Egg size 67–71 x 44–45 μm.

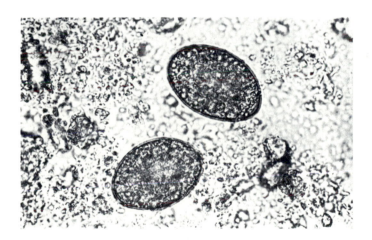

FIG. 1.113.   Eggs of *Dibothriocephalus latus*. ×410.

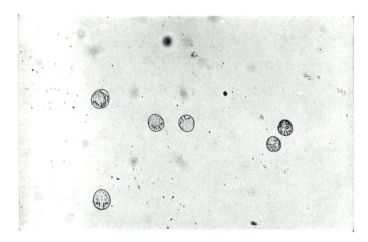

FIG. 1.114.   Eggs of *Mesocestoides variabilis,* a seldom-reported tapeworm of dogs, foxes, cats, and rarely of man; also of coyotes, lynxes, opossums, raccoons, and skunks. These eggs were removed from the egg sac of a ripe segment. ×100. Egg size 20–25 µm in diameter.

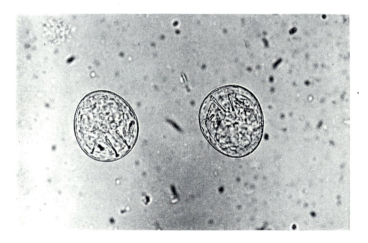

FIG. 1.115.   Eggs of *Mesocestoides variabilis.* ×410.

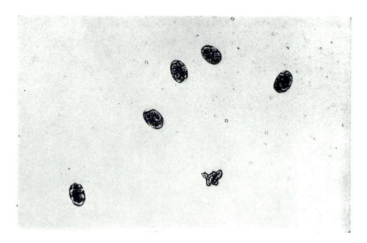

FIG. 1.116. Eggs of *Ancylostoma caninum*, the more common hookworm of dogs, foxes, and coyotes. ×100. Egg size 56–65 x 37–43 μm.

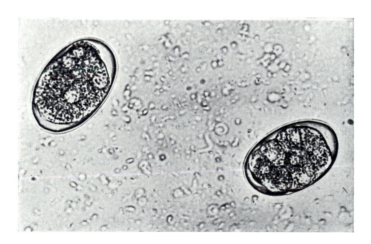

FIG. 1.117. Eggs of *Ancylostoma caninum*. Eggs are observed in various stages of segmentation. ×410.

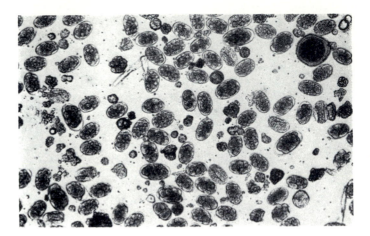

FIG. 1.118.   Eggs of *Uncinaria stenocephala* (larger eggs), hookworm of dogs, cats, foxes, and wolves, and of *Ancylostoma caninum* (smaller eggs), hookworm of dogs, foxes, and wolves. *A. tubaeforme* of cats has a similar egg. At the upper right is an egg of *Toxocara canis,* one of the ascarids (see Figs. 1.120, 1.121). ×100. *Uncinaria* egg size 65–80 x 40-50 μm; *Ancylostoma* egg size 56–65 x 37-43 μm.

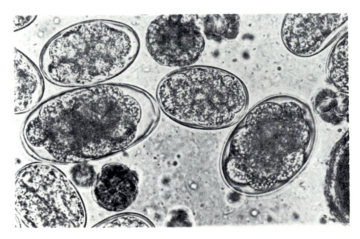

FIG. 1.119.   Eggs of *Uncinaria stenocephala* (larger eggs) and *Ancylostoma caninum* (smaller eggs). ×410.

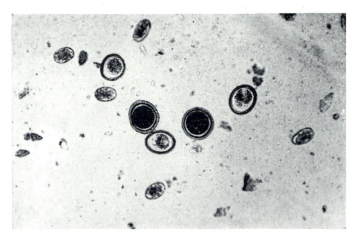

FIG. 1.120.   Eggs of *Toxocara canis* and *Toxascaris leonina*, both species of ascarids of dogs, foxes, and coyotes; also occur in cats, bobcats, and wolves. Included are five eggs of *Ancylostoma caninum*, a hookworm of dogs, foxes, and coyotes. ×100. *Toxocara* egg size 90 x 75 μm; *Toxascaris* egg size 75–85 x 60–75 μm.

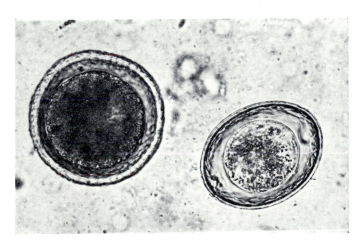

FIG. 1.121.   Eggs of *Toxocara canis (left)* and *Toxascaris leonina (right)*. ×410.

Note: *Toxocara canis* egg is yellowish brown with crinkled or pitted shell. *Toxascaris leonina* egg is colorless with smooth shell.

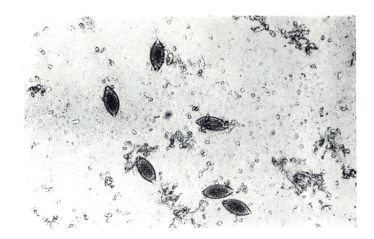

FIG. 1.122.   Eggs of *Trichuris vulpis,* the whipworm of dogs, foxes, and coyotes.   × 100. Egg size 70–89 x 37–40 μm.

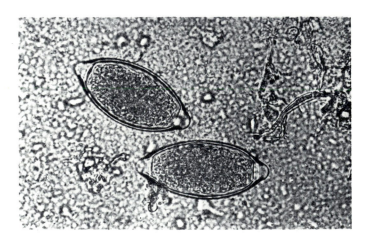

FIG. 1.123.   Eggs of *Trichuris vulpis.* Note the larger size and smooth shell compared with lungworm eggs (see Fig. 1.127).   ×410.

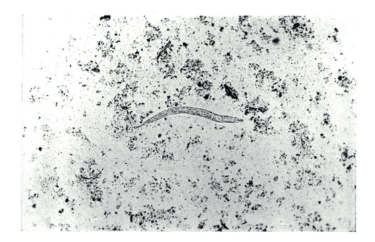

FIG. 1.124. Rhabditiform larva of *Strongyloides stercoralis*, the threadworm of dogs, foxes, cats, and probably of man. The eggs hatch in the intestinal mucosa. ×100.

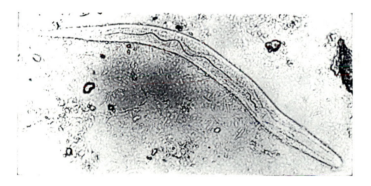

FIG. 1.125. Rhabditiform larva of *Strongyloides stercoralis*. ×410.

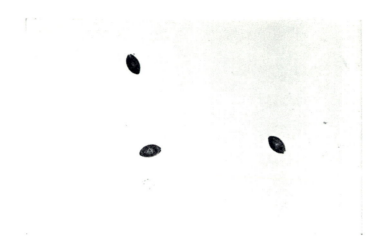

FIG. 1.126. Eggs of *Capillaria aerophila*, the most common lungworm of dogs, cats, and foxes. ×100. Egg size 59–80 x 30–40 μm.

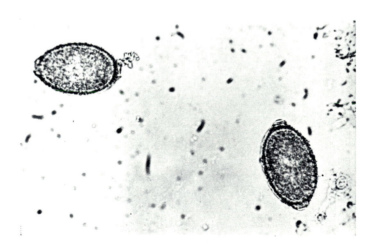

FIG. 1.127. Eggs of *Capillaria aerophila*. The color is yellowish. The shells are finely granular, and there is a plug at each end. The size and granular shell differentiate them from eggs of *Trichuris vulpis,* the whipworm (Fig. 1.123). ×410.

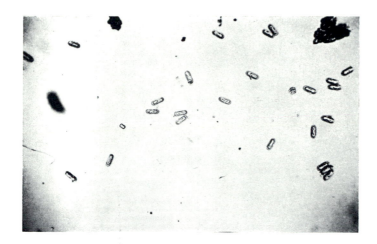

FIG. 1.128.   Eggs of *Spirocerca lupi,* the esophageal worm of dogs and foxes; also of bobcats and wolves. ×100. Egg size 30–37 x 11–15 μm.

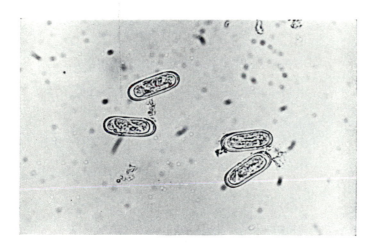

FIG. 1.129.   Eggs of *Spirocerca lupi.* These eggs are embryonated when laid. ×410.

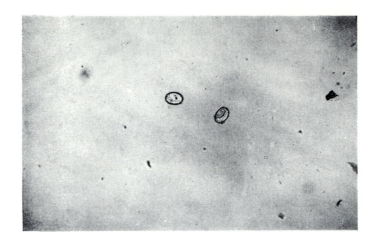

FIG. 1.130.   Eggs of *Physaloptera rara*, a stomach worm of dogs, cats, and foxes; also of bobcats, coyotes, raccoons, and wolves. × 100. Egg size 40 x 34 μm.

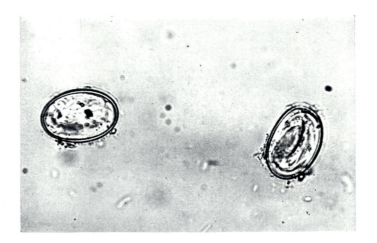

FIG. 1.131.   Eggs of *Physaloptera rara*. These eggs are embryonated when laid. × 410.

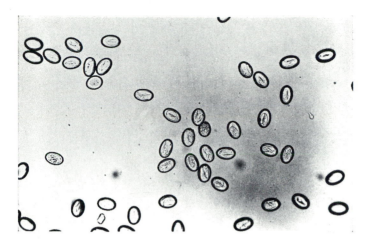

FIG. 1.132.   Eggs of *Physaloptera praeputialis,* a stomach worm of dogs, cats, and foxes; also of bobcats, coyotes, lynxes, and mountain lions. × 100. Egg size 49–58 x 30–34 μm.

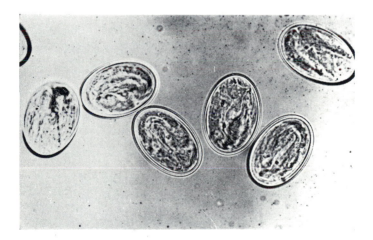

FIG. 1.133.   Eggs of *Physaloptera praeputialis.* These eggs are embryonated when laid. × 410.

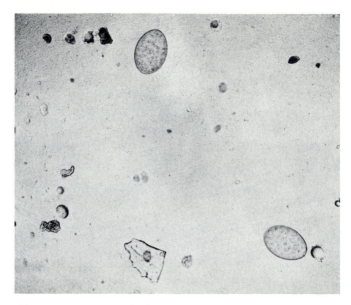

FIG. 1.134.   Eggs of *Alaria canis,* an intestinal fluke. The eggs are yellow, thin-shelled, and partially embryonated. × 100. Egg size 117–126 x 74–78 µm.

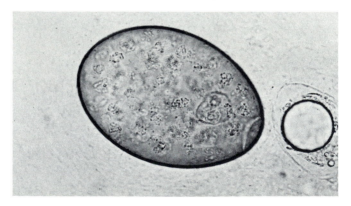

FIG. 1.135.   *Alaria canis* egg. × 410.

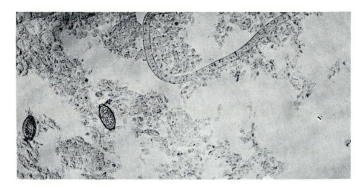

FIG. 1.136. *Capillaria plica* eggs and larva. This is a parasite of the urinary bladder, but the eggs are frequently found in the feces. × 100. Egg size 63–68 x 24–27 μm.

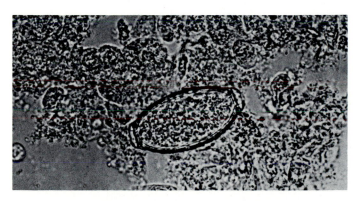

FIG. 1.137. *Capillaria plica* egg. × 410.

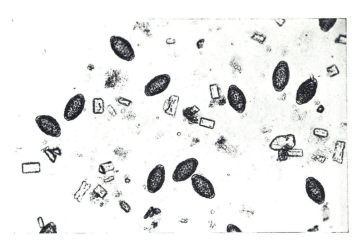

FIG. 1.138.   Eggs of *Dioctophyma renale,* the giant kidney worm of dogs, foxes, and rarely of man; also of coyotes, minks, otters, raccoons, weasels, wolves, and wolverines. These eggs are usually found in urinary sediment (note triple phosphate crystals). They may also be found in feces contaminated by urine. × 100. Egg size 71–84 x 46–52 μm.

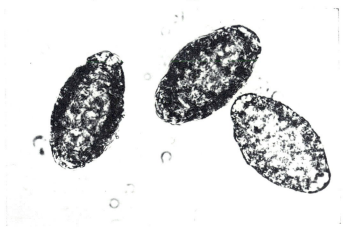

FIG. 1.139.   Eggs of *Dioctophyma renale.* The shells are thick and rough and yellowish brown. × 410.

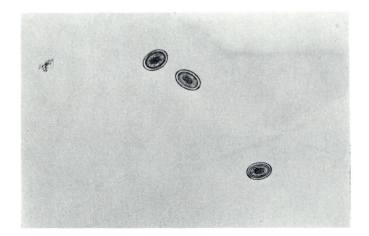

FIG. 1.140.   Eggs of *Oncicola canis,* the thorny-headed worm of dogs, cats, and coyotes.   ×100.   Egg size 59–71 x 40–50 μm.

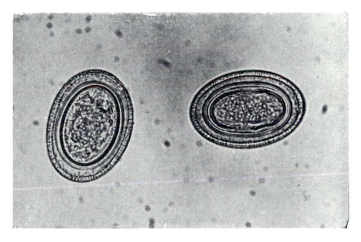

FIG. 1.141.   Eggs of *Oncicola canis.* Note the three shells enclosing the embryo.   ×410.

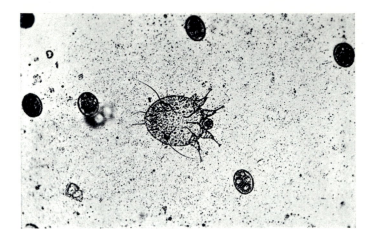

FIG. 1.142.   A larva of *Sarcoptes scabiei* var. *canis,* the sarcoptic mange mite of dogs. Also shown are several eggs of *Ancylostoma caninum,* a hookworm, in dog feces. Mange, especially in dogs and cats, may be diagnosed by fecal examination if the host happens to ingest mites when biting the skin lesions. ×100.

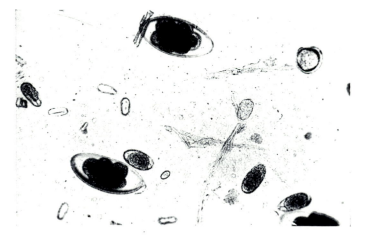

FIG.   1.143.   Spurious parasites. The feces of this dog contain eggs and oocysts of sheep parasites. The dog's food was contaminated by sheep feces. The field contains eggs of *Nematodirus   spathiger,   Moniezia   expansa,* and *Strongyloides papillosus* and an unidentified nematode egg and a coccidial oocyst. ×100.

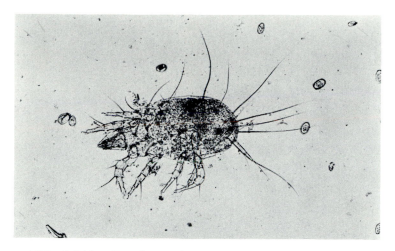

FIG. 1.144. Pseudoparasite. An adult "grain" mite and coccidial oocysts in the feces of a dog. ×100.

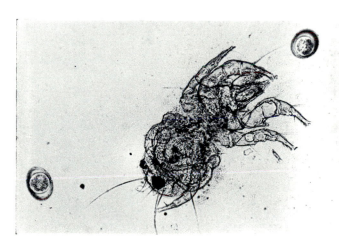

FIG. 1.145. Pseudoparasite. An adult "grain" mite and two eggs of *Toxascaris leonina* in dog feces. ×100.

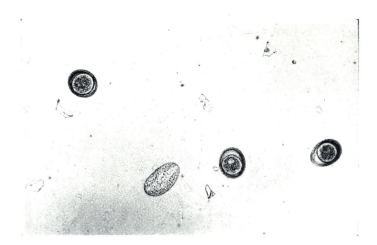

FIG. 1.146.   Pseudoparasite. An egg of a "grain" mite and three eggs of *Toxascaris leonina* in dog feces. ×100.

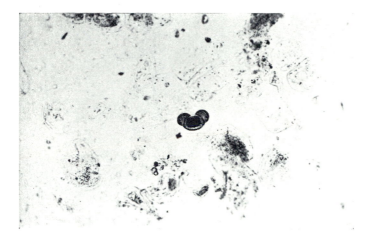

FIG. 1.147. Pseudoparasite. Pine pollen in dog feces. The color is pale brown. ×100.

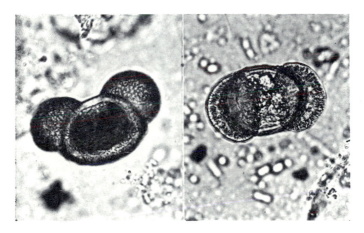

FIG. 1.148. Pine pollen in the feces of a dog. Side view of a pollen grain *(left)*, showing the two winglike floats; *(right)* view from above. ×410.

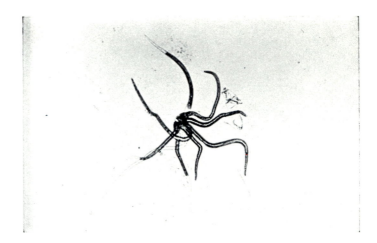

FIG. 1.149.   Pseudoparasite. Plant hairs from dog feces. These resemble the groups of hairlike projections seen on the under surface of oak leaves. ×100.

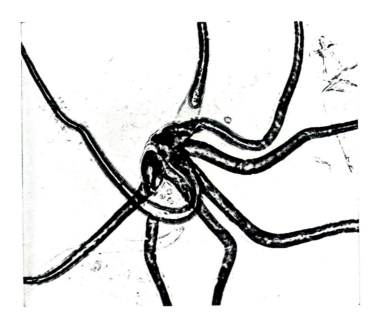

FIG. 1.150.   Plant hairs from dog feces. ×338.

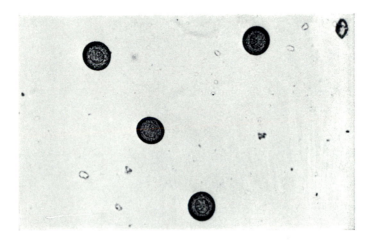

FIG. 1.151. Spurious parasite. The feces of this dog contained eggs of *Hymenolepis diminuta,* a tapeworm of rats, mice, and man. Presumably the dog ingested the small intestine of an infected rodent. These eggs are yellow in color. ×100. Egg size 60–80 x 72–86 μm.

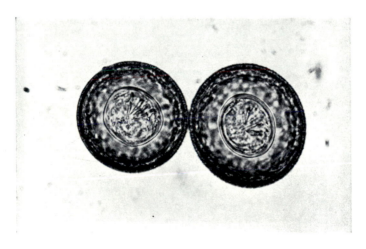

FIG. 1.152. *Hymenolepis diminuta* eggs in dog feces. Note the six hooklets in each embryo. ×410.

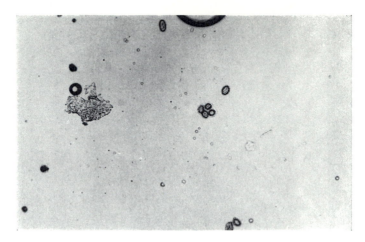

FIG. 1.153. Pseudoparasite. Corn smut spores in the feces of a dog. These resemble certain tapeworm eggs under low magnification. ×100.

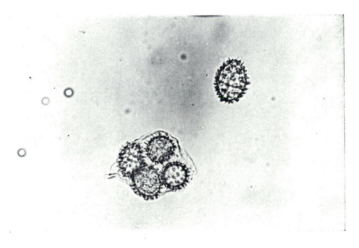

FIG. 1.154. Corn smut spores in feces. Note the spiny covering. ×410.

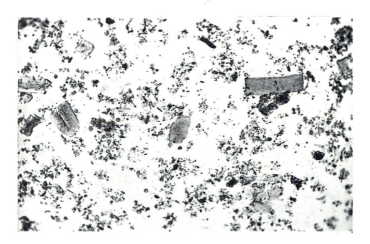

FIG. 1.155.   Undigested muscle in a dog's feces. ×100.

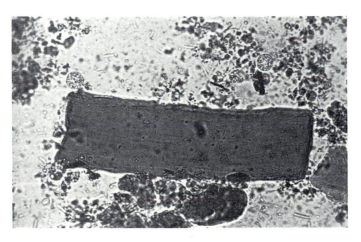

FIG. 1.156.   Undigested muscle in a dog's feces. ×410.

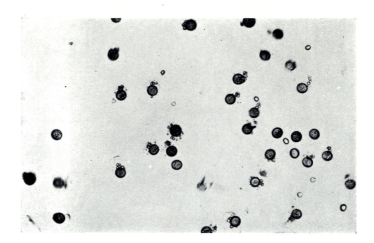

FIG. 1.157.   Eggs of *Hydatigera taeniaeformis,* a common tapeworm of cats and bobcats. × 100. Egg size 31 x 37 μm.

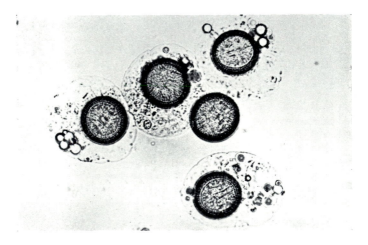

FIG. 1.158.   Eggs of *Hydatigera taeniaeformis.* Four of these are enclosed in embryonic membranes. × 410.

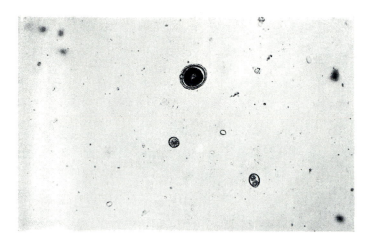

FIG. 1.159. Egg of *Toxocara mystax,* an ascarid of cats; also found in bobcats and lynxes. Also shown are two oocysts of a coccidium, *Isospora felis* (see Note, p. 68). × 100. Egg size 65 x 75 μm. Oocyst size 32–53 x 26–43 μm.

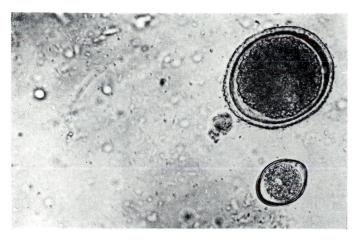

FIG. 1.160. Egg of *Toxocara mystax* and an oocyst of *Isospora felis.* × 410.

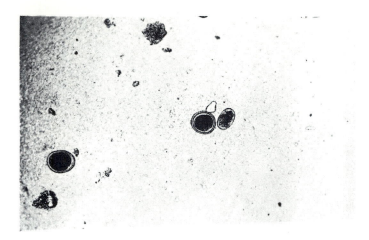

FIG. 1.161.   Eggs of *Toxocara mystax,* an ascarid of cats; also found in bobcats and lynxes. Also shown is an egg of *Ancylostoma tubaeforme.* ×100. *Toxocara mystax* egg size 65 x 75   μm.   *Ancylostoma   tubaeforme   egg   size* 55–76 x 34–45 μm.

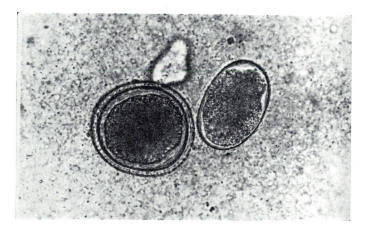

FIG. 1.162.   Egg of *Toxocara mystax* and egg of *Ancylostoma tubaeforme.* ×410.

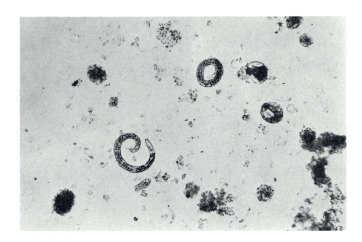

FIG. 1.163. Eggs and larvae of *Aelurostrongylus abstrusus*, the lungworm of cats. ×100. Egg size 80 x 70 μm.

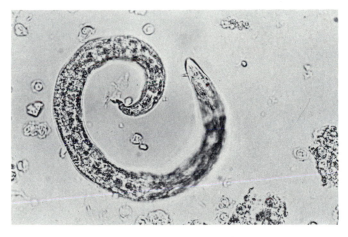

FIG. 1.164. Larva of *Aelurostrongylus abstrusus*. Note the characteristic kinked tail. ×410.

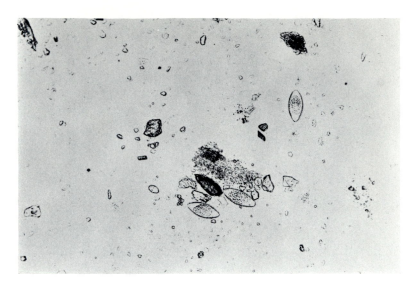

FIG. 1.165.   Eggs of *Aspiculuris tetraptera*, the pinworm of rodents. × 100. Egg size 20–98 x 29–50 μm.

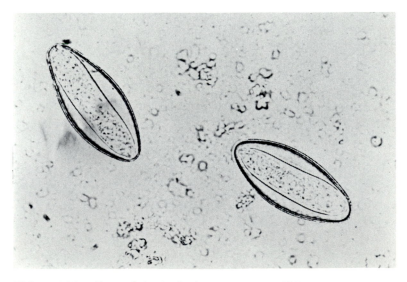

FIG. 1.166.   Eggs of *Aspiculuris tetraptera*. × 400.

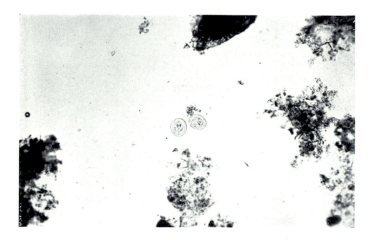

FIG. 1.167. Eggs of *Hymenolepis nana*, the dwarf tapeworm of man, rats, and mice. ×100. Egg size 30 x 47 μm in diameter.

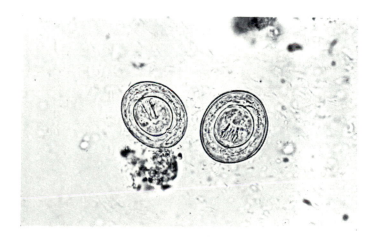

FIG. 1.168. Eggs of *Hymenolepis nana*. There are four to eight slender filaments on each polar thickening of the inner shell membrane. ×385.

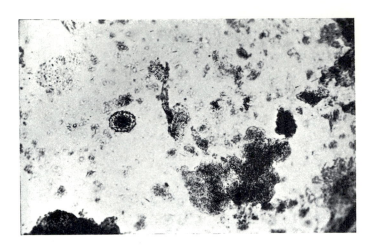

FIG. 1.169.   Egg of *Ascaris lumbricoides,* the ascarid of man. × 100. Egg size 50–75 x 40–50 μm.

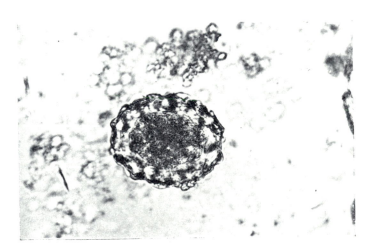

FIG. 1.170.   Egg of *Ascaris lumbricoides.* × 410.

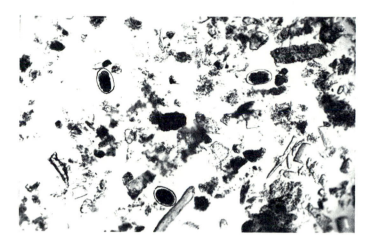

FIG. 1.171.   Eggs of *Necator americanus*, the new-world hookworm of man. Simple smear.   ×100. Egg size 64–76 x 36–40 μm.

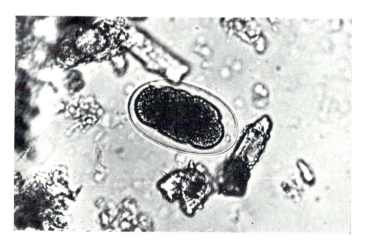

FIG. 1.172.   Egg of *Necator americanus*. ×410.

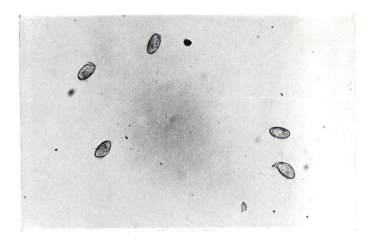

FIG. 1.173. Eggs of *Enterobius vermicularis*, the pinworm or rectal worm of man. × 100. Egg size 50-60 x 20-30 μm.

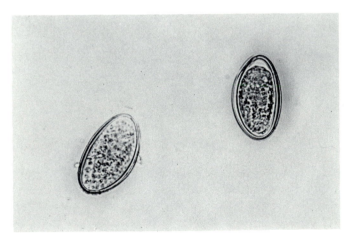

FIG. 1.174.   Eggs of *Enterobius vermicularis*. × 410.

*Note: The dog does **not** have a pinworm.*

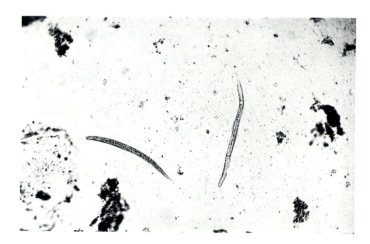

FIG. 1.175. Larvae of *Strongyloides stercoralis,* the threadworm of man. ×100.

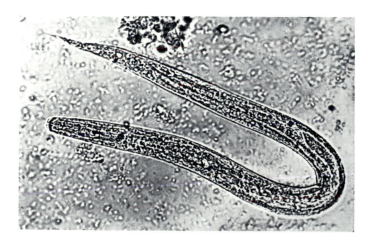

FIG. 1.176. Larva of *Strongyloides stercoralis.* ×410.

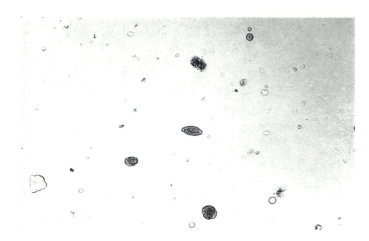

FIG. 1.177.   Egg of *Trichuris trichiura*, the whipworm of man. ×100. Egg size 50-60 x 21-25 µm.

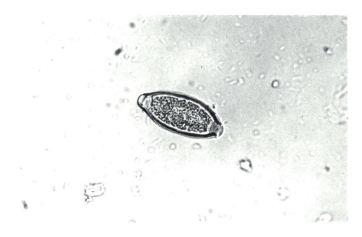

FIG. 1.178.   Egg of *Trichuris trichiura*. Note the resemblance to the eggs of the swine whipworm (Fig. 1.89). ×410.

FIG. 1.179.   Eggs of *Taenia saginata,* the beef tapeworm of man. ×100. Egg size 30-50 x 20-30 μm.

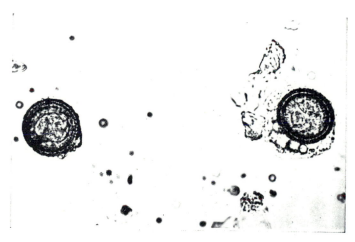

FIG. 1.180.   Eggs of *Taenia saginata.* The egg at right is contained within an embryonic membrane. ×410.

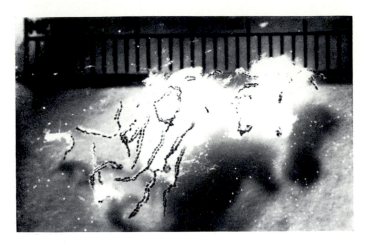

FIG. 1.181. Pseudoparasite. Banana seeds in human feces. Grossly these resemble small brownish tapeworm segments. ×3.

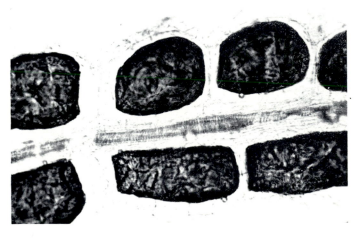

FIG. 1.182. Banana seeds in human feces. ×100.

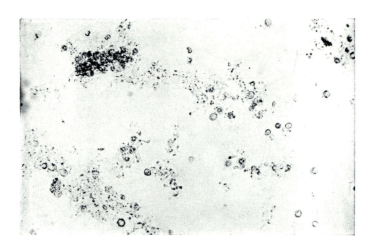

FIG. 1.183.   Oocysts of *Eimeria tenella,* the cecal coccidium of chickens. × 100. Oocyst size 14–31 x 9–25 μm.

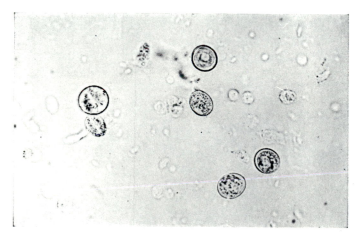

FIG. 1.184.   Oocysts of *Eimeria tenella.* × 410.

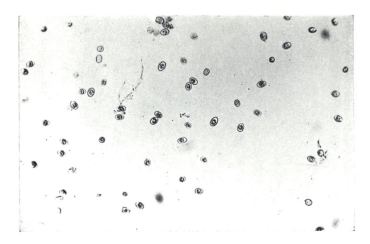

FIG. 1.185. Oocysts of *Eimeria meleagridis* and *Eimeria meleagrimitis*, two species of coccidia of turkeys. ×100. Oocyst size 16–27 x 13–22 μm.

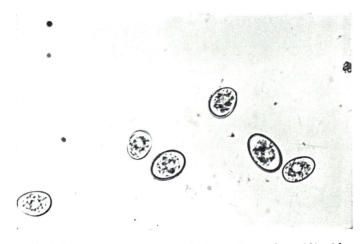

FIG. 1.186. Two oocysts of *Eimeria meleagridis* (the larger ones) and four oocysts of *Eimeria meleagrimitis*. ×410.

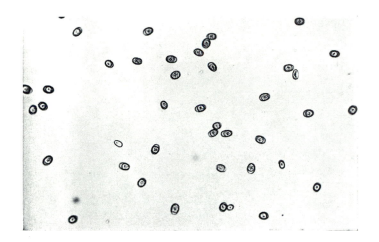

FIG. 1.187.   Oocysts of *Eimeria dispersa* and *Eimeria pha-siani,* coccidia of pheasants.   ×100.   Oocyst size 22–31 x 18–24 μm.

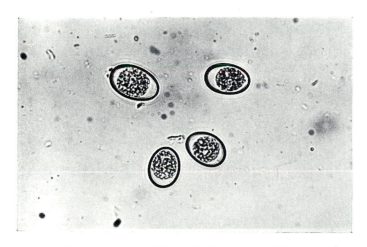

FIG. 1.188.   Oocysts of *Eimeria dispersa* and *Eimeria pha-siani.* The latter are slightly larger. ×410.

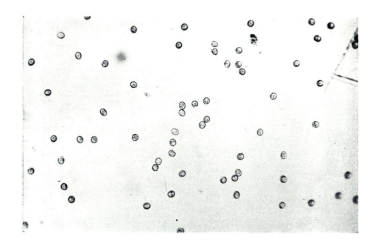

FIG. 1.189.   Oocysts of *Eimeria labbeana,* the coccidium of pigeons. ×100. Oocyst size 13–24 x 12–23 µm.

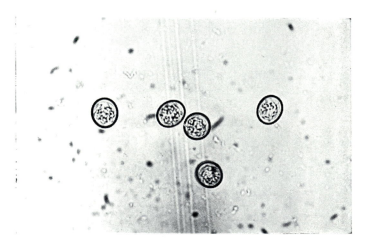

FIG. 1.190.   Oocysts of *Eimeria labbeana.* ×410.

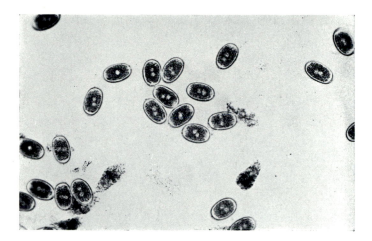

FIG. 1.191. Eggs of *Ascaridia galli*, the ascarid of chickens and rarely of turkeys and guinea fowl; also of prairie chickens and sharp-tailed grouse. ×100. Egg size 73–92 x 45–57 μm.

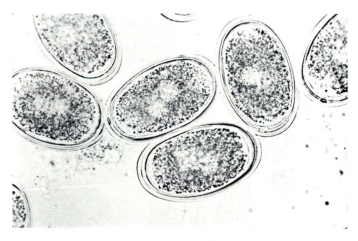

FIG. 1.192.   Eggs of *Ascaridia galli*. ×400.

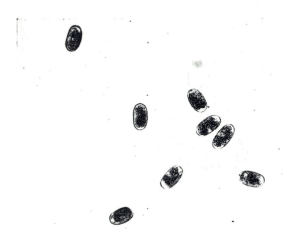

FIG. 1.193.   Eggs of *Heterakis gallinarum,* the cecal worm of chickens, turkeys, and guinea fowl; also of partridges, pheasants, prairie chickens, quail, and grouse. ×100. Egg size 65–80 x 35–46 μm.

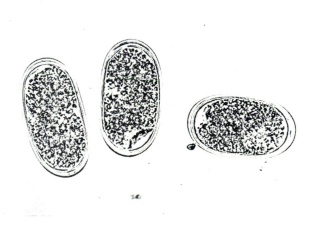

FIG. 1.194.   Eggs of *Heterakis gallinarum.* ×410.

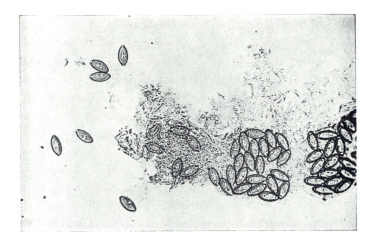

FIG. 1.195. Eggs of *Capillaria contorta*, the crop capillarid of chickens, turkeys, ducks, grouse, quail, and pheasants. ×100. Egg size 48–56 x 21–24 μm.

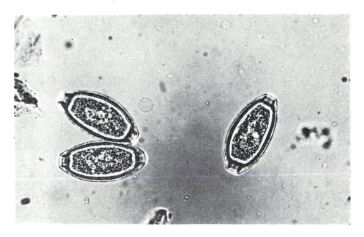

FIG. 1.196. Eggs of *Capillaria contorta*. Note the plug at each pole. ×410.

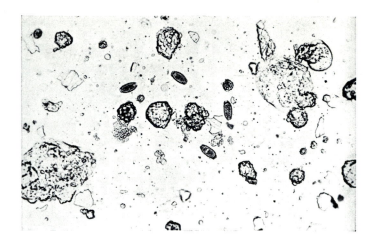

FIG. 1.197.   Eggs of *Capillaria caudinflata,* a capillarid worm of the small intestine of chickens, turkeys, and pheasants. ×100. Egg size 60–65 x 23 μm.

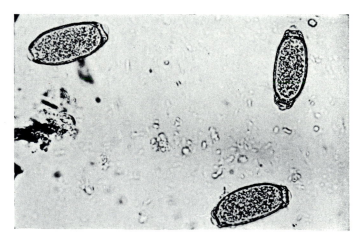

FIG. 1.198.   Eggs of *Capillaria caudinflata.* Note the plug at each pole. ×410.

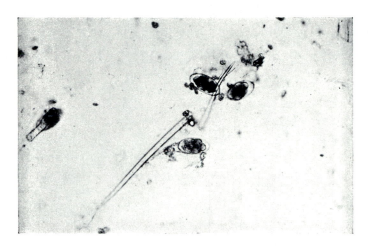

FIG. 1.199.   Eggs of *Syngamus trachea,* the gapeworm of chickens, turkeys, and guinea fowl; also of crows, grackles, grouse, juncos, meadowlarks, partridges, pheasants, quail, robins, sparrows, and thrushes.   ×100.   Egg size 78–110 x 43–46 μm.

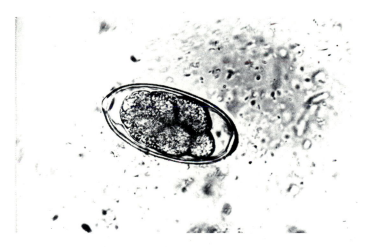

FIG. 1.200.   Egg of *Syngamus trachea.* Note the operculum at each pole. ×410.

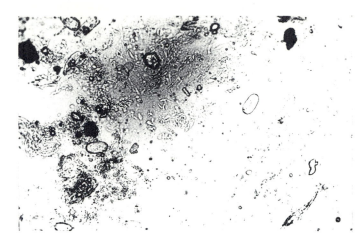

FIG. 1.201.   Eggs of *Tetrameres americana*, the globular stomach worm of chickens, pigeons, and quail. ×100. Egg size 42–50 x 25 µm.

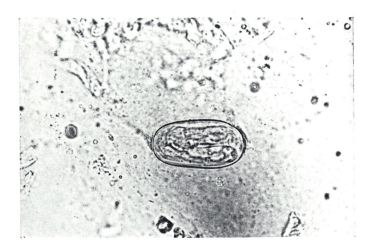

FIG. 1.202.   Egg of *Tetrameres americana*. The eggs of this nematode are embryonated when laid. ×410.

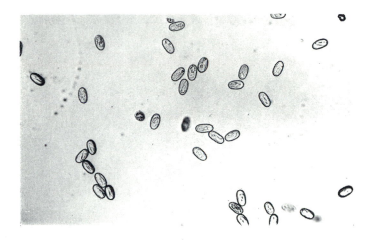

FIG. 1.203. Eggs of *Dispharynx nasuta,* the spiral stomach worm of chickens, turkeys, guinea fowl, and pigeons; also of grouse, partridges, pheasants, and quail. ×100. Egg size 33–40 x 18–25 μm.

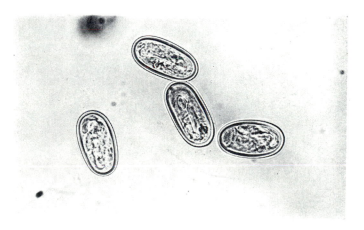

FIG. 1.204. Eggs of *Dispharynx nasuta*. The eggs are embryonated when laid. ×410.

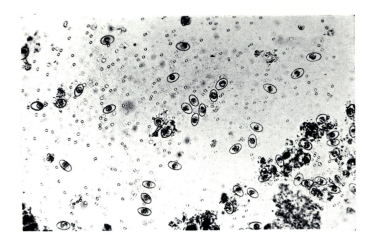

FIG. 1.205.   Oocysts of *Eimeria stiedai*, the hepatic coccidium of rabbits and hares. These were removed from the
bile duct. They may also be found in the feces. × 100.
Oocyst size 28–40 x 16–25 μm.

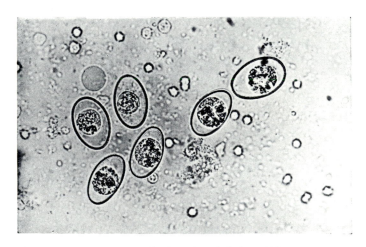

FIG. 1.206.   Oocysts of *Eimeria stiedai*. × 410.

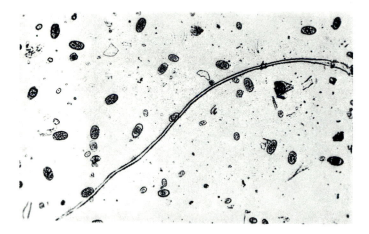

FIG. 1.207. Oocysts of several *Eimeria* species, intestinal coccidia of rabbits. A long plant hair is present. × 100.

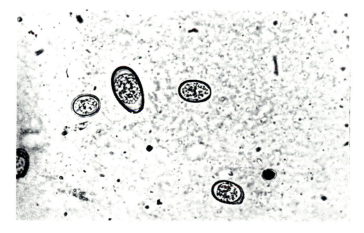

FIG. 1.208. Oocysts of three *Eimeria* species. × 410.

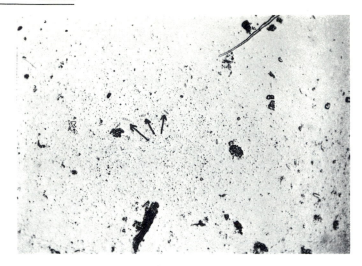

FIG. 1.209. Pseudoparasite. *Saccharomycopsis guttulatus,* a yeast commonly found in the feces of rabbits, chinchillas, and guinea pigs. It is believed to be non-pathogenic. Arrows point to the yeasts. × 100.

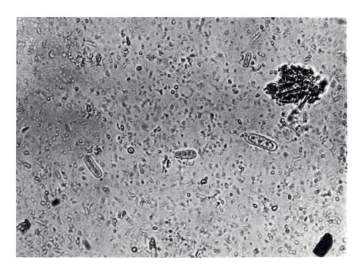

FIG. 1.210. Pseudoparasite. *Saccharomycopsis guttulatus.* × 410.

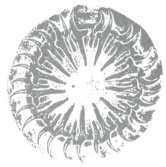

Section Two

PARASITES OF THE BLOOD

The blood of domesticated animals may be invaded by various pathogenic and nonpathogenic microorganisms such as bacteria, viruses, rickettsiae, fungi, and yeasts. Also certain parasitic members of the *animal* kingdom invade the blood, either for a primary location or as a means of transport to other body structures where they complete their development. These animal parasites include numerous species of protozoa, a few species of adult and larval flukes, occasionally larval tapeworms, several species of adult and larval nematodes, and, rarely, the adult and immature stages of mites.

Some parasites reach the blood actively by penetration through the skin or mucous membranes. Others are introduced passively through wounds caused by foreign bodies; by helminths; by the bites of insects, mites, and ticks; or through surface tissues damaged by chemicals of bacterial or other origins.

The domesticated animal hosts to be considered will include those of continental North America north of Mexico: horses, cattle, sheep, swine, dogs, cats, and domesticated poultry. Parasites will be briefly described under three groups: protozoa, nematodes, and mites. This will be followed by concise directions for their laboratory identification.

The dimensions of microscopic parasites may be determined by means of a micrometer disk inserted in the ocular of a microscope (see pp. 3–5, Section One, for calibration instructions). Or a separate micrometer-ocular may be used for the most accurate measuring. If a micrometer is not available, the size of a microscopic parasite may be approximated by comparing it with the dimensions of the erythrocytes as seen in properly stained blood-film preparations.

TABLE 2.1.   Average Diameters of Erythrocytes*

Horse — 5.7 μm	Dog — 7.0 μm
Cattle — 5.6 μm	Cat — 5.9 μm
Sheep — 5.0 μm	Chicken — 12.3 x 6.9 μm
Goat — 4.3 μm	Turkey — 11.2 x 6.4 μm
Swine — 6.1 μm	Birds (46 species) — 13-15 x 7.5 μm

*Measurements from Scarborough 1930-32, with the exception of the turkey (West and Starr 1940), and the chicken (Lucas and Jamroz, 1961).

PROTOZOA AND RICKETTSIAE

Most of the protozoan and rickettsial parasites that invade the blood are destructive to erythrocytes. Hence, when patients show clinical symptoms of anemia, their blood should be examined for hemoglobin content and for cellular numbers. Carefully prepared blood films should then be examined for the presence of erythrocytes having abnormal size, shape, and poor staining reaction. Also the cells and the plasma should be searched for evidence of parasites.

Anaplasma marginale, anaplasmosis organism of cattle, deer. More or less spherical bodies in erythrocytes, about 90% being located marginally. To 0.8 μm in diameter (Figs. 2.3, 2.4).

Anaplasma ovis, anaplasmosis organism of sheep. More or less spherical bodies in erythrocytes, about 60% being located marginally. To 0.8 μm in diameter.

Babesia bigemina, southern cattle fever piroplasm of cattle. Ovoid to conoidal bodies — singly, in pairs, or multiple — in erythrocytes. 2.5-5.5 (av. 4.02) μm long x 2 μm wide. Average angle of pairs is 57 degrees (Fig. 2.5).

Babesia argentina, "Argentine" cattle fever piroplasm of cattle. Ovoid to conoidal bodies — singly, in pairs, or multiple — in erythrocytes. 2-4.5 (av. 3.14) μm long x 2 μm wide. Average angle of pairs is 129.9 degrees.

Babesia canis, piroplasmosis organism of dog. Spherical to conoidal bodies — singly, in pairs, or multiple — in erythrocytes. 4.5-5 μm long (Fig. 2.6).

Eperythrozoon wenyoni, eperythrozoonosis organism of cattle. Typically delicate ring-forms on the surface of erythrocytes or in plasma. 0.3–1.5 μm in diameter.

Eperythrozoon sp., eperythrozoonosis organism of sheep. Typically delicate ring-forms on the surface of erythrocytes or in plasma. 0.3–1.5 μm in diameter.

Eperythrozoon suis, eperythrozoonosis organism of swine. Typically delicate ring-forms on the surface of erythrocytes or in plasma. 0.8–2.5 μm in diameter.

Eperythrozoon parvum, nonpathogenic (?) eperythrozoonosis organism of swine. Mostly spherical (coccoid) forms on the surface of erythrocytes. Some ring-forms seen. Spherical forms less than 0.5 μm, ring-forms about 0.5 μm in diameter.

Gonderia mutans (= Theileria mutans), gonderiosis organism of cattle. One or more bodies in erythrocytes, shaped like cocci, rods, rings, commas, dumbbells, or crosses. Diameter or length to 2 μm.

Haemobartonella bovis, haemobartonellosis organism of cattle. Spherical bodies, usually paired, rodlike forms on the erythrocytes and occasionally in plasma. About 2 μm in diameter.

Haemobartonella canis, haemobartonellosis organism of dog. Spherical, ovoid, and rod-shaped bodies — singly or in chains — on erythrocytes and occasionally in plasma. Spherical and ovoid forms 0.2–0.4 μm in diameter, rods to 6 μm long.

Haemobartonella felis, haemobartonellosis (feline infectious anemia) organism of cat. Spherical, ovoid, rod-shaped, and occasionally ringlike bodies on erythrocytes and occasionally in plasma. Spherical forms 0.2–0.3 μm in diameter, rods 0.7–0.9 μm long with average diameter about 0.3 μm.

Haemoproteus meleagridis, haemoproteosis organism of turkey. A cylindrical, crescentic, blood-pigmented body with rounded ends in the cytoplasm of erythrocytes. Adult female gametocytes 13.94–19.39 μm long and 2.42–4.24 μm wide, occupying one-half to three-fourths of the cytoplasm; adult male gametocytes 13.03–17.81 μm long x 2.88–3.94 μm wide.

Haemoproteus nettionis, haemoproteosis organism of ducks and geese, both domesticated and wild. A cylindrical, blood-pigmented body with rounded ends in the cytoplasm of erythrocytes, often pushing the nucleus to one side. Adult female gametocytes 13–28 μm long x 2–3.5 μm wide; adult male gametocytes 14–28 μm long x 2–5 μm wide.

Haemoproteus columbae, haemoproteosis organism of pigeons, doves. A cylindrical, blood-pigmented body with rounded ends in the cytoplasm of erythrocytes, partly or completely surrounding the nucleus which may be displaced laterally. Adult female and male gametocytes about 8 μm long x 1–2 μm wide (Fig. 2.7).

Haemoproteus sacharovi, haemoproteosis organism of pigeons, doves. Morphology similar to *Haemoproteus columbae* except (1) there is little pigment in the parasites and (2) as they develop within the erythrocytes, the latter show a distinct tendency to become swolien (hypertrophy?). Measurements not given in the literature consulted.

Leucocytozoon (Akiba) caulleryi, leucocytozoonosis organism (rarely reported) of chicken presumably in leukocytes and erythrocytes. Adult female gametocyte spherical, averaging 12–14 μm in diameter, distending the host cell and pushing its nucleus to one side; adult male gametocyte spherical, averaging 10–12 μm in diameter.

Leucocytozoon (Leucocytozoon) smithi, leucocytozoonosis organism of turkey presumably in leukocytes or possibly in erythrocytes, although Johnson (1942) considers the parasites (gametocytes) to be free in the blood plasma. Spherical to ovoid to spindle-shaped masses containing one to four elongated, deeply staining structures (called host-cell nuclei by some and lateral bars by others). Female 19.18–23.18 μm long (West and Starr 1940); male 18.31–23.89 μm long (Fig. 2.8).

Leucocytozoon (Leucocytozoon) simondi, leucocytozoonosis organism of domesticated and wild ducks and wild geese. Types of blood cells invaded are not definitely determined. Cook (1954) considered them to be members of the erythrocytic series (reticulocytes and erythrocytes). Young parasites (gametocytes) first appear as ringlike forms having a diameter of 1 μm when in reticulocytes and lymphocytes. More mature forms in erythrocytes are rounded, having diameters of 10–16 μm. Later, spindle-shaped forms appear in the greatly enlarged host cells.

Plasmodium (Haemamoeba) relictum, a malaria organism of pigeons, doves, and many wild birds. The erythrocyte-invading form of the parasite begins with the entrance of a minute body (merozoite) which soon becomes ringlike, 1–2 μm in diameter. This grows (trophozoite) to later become a form (schizont) that distends, almost fills, and eventually destroys the erythrocyte, liberating many reinfective forms (merozoites). Later certain merozoites invade erythrocytes to develop into female or male parasites (gametocytes), which almost fill and then destroy the cells. The larger forms of *P. relictum* contain relatively fine, spherical blood pigment granules.

Trypanosoma equiperdum, trypanosome of dourine of horses and donkeys. Dourine is now nearly eradicated in North America. The organism occurs in blood plasma. It is elongated, tapers at both ends, and has a single flagellum anteriorly that is seen as a continuation of a long, lateral undulating membrane. 25–30 μm long x 1–2 μm wide (Fig. 2.9).

Trypanosoma theileri, a relatively nonpathogenic trypanosome of cattle. Rather frequently seen in small numbers in bovine blood plasma in smears or in hemocytometer chambers. This trypanosome tapers at both ends and has an undulating membrane extending along the anterior third of the body and continued by a long flagellum. 14–40 μm x 3.8–5 μm. Total length including flagellum may be 75 μm.

Trypanosoma melophagium, nonpathogenic trypanosome of sheep. Rarely seen in blood plasma. It is a common inhabitant of the digestive tract of the sheep "tick" fly or ked *(Melophagus ovinus;* see Fig. 5.12). This trypanosome is elongated, tapers at both ends, and has a short anterior flagellum continuous with a rudimentary type of undulating membrane. 50–60 μm long.

Toxoplasma gondii, toxoplasmosis organism of all domesticated and many wild animal hosts and man. This organism is present in blood plasma only during its dissemination to the many organs and tissues in which it undergoes multiplication. It is a protozoon closely related to *Sarcocystis* and to coccidia of the genus *Isospora*. Individual organisms are crescentic, 6-7 μm long x 3-4 μm wide (Fig. 2.10).

NEMATODE LARVAE

Many species of parasitic worms enter the blood stream of the host in order to reach certain organs or tissues where they develop to maturity. Their stay in the blood is usually only minutes or hours, hence they are seldom seen in blood specimens taken for diagnostic purposes.

However, there is a group of related nematodes (filariids) whose larvae (microfilariae) are, of necessity, found in the circulation. Here they wait for the arrival of their blood-sucking intermediate hosts, in which they must undergo further development to an inoculative stage. These intermediate hosts are blood-sucking insects.

The following nematodes include those filariids whose microfilariae may be seen during microscopic examination of the blood.

Dirofilaria immitis, heartworm of dog, cat, fox, coyote, wolf. The adult heartworms are found in the right atrium, right ventricle, pulmonary artery, and erratically in the lungs, bronchioles, peritoneal cavity, and eyes. Adult heartworms about 1 mm in diameter; females 25-30 cm long, males 12-18 cm long. The larvae in peripheral blood plasma are 307-322 μm long x 6.7-7.1 μm wide, and their posterior ends are mostly straight when fixed in 2% formaldehyde solution (Figs. 2.13-2.17).

Dipetalonema reconditum, subcutaneous worm of dog. Larvae in peripheral blood plasma are 269-283 μm long x 4.3-4.8 μm wide, and their posterior ends are curved ("button-hook") when fixed in 2% formaldehyde solution.

Ornithofilaria fallisensis, subcutaneous worm of ducks—both domesticated and wild—and wild geese. Larvae in peripheral blood plasma are 50-121 μm long.

Setaria cervi, peritoneal worm of cattle. The *sheathed* larvae are in the plasma of the peripheral blood. Their length is usually given as 140-230 μm. Bell (1934) stated that the microfilariae including the sheath average 312 x 9.02 μm and the microfilariae not including the sheath average 280 x 6.92 μm.

Setaria equina, peritoneal worm of horse. The *sheathed* larvae are in peripheral blood plasma. Reported size averages 280 μm long x 7 μm wide (Figs. 2.11, 2.12).

MITES
Mites are usually parasites of the skin and adjacent structures. Several species of mites regularly invade internal organs: air sacs, pneumatic bone cavities, and subcutis of birds; nasal cavities and paranasal sinuses of dogs; and the auditory canals of horses, cattle, sheep, dogs, and cats.

Apparently the only record of mites found in the bloodstream of domesticated animals is that by Koutz (1957), who reported the occurrence of demodectic mange mites in the internal organs of dogs.

Demodex canis, demodectic mange mite of dog. Koutz (1957) found larvae, nymphs, and adults in the blood of 20% of dogs having demodectic mange. Mites were also found in lymph nodes, spleen, kidneys (and urine), and intestines (and feces). It is not known if the mites actually reproduce in the bloodstream or are simply using the blood of the host as a means of transport. Reported measurements for female *Demodex canis* are 180–302 μm long x 45 μm wide (see Fig. 3.55); for males, 220–250 μm long x 45 μm wide; for larvae, 140 μm long x 40 μm wide; and for nymphs, 180 μm long x 50 μm wide (Neveu-Lemaire 1943).

LABORATORY IDENTIFICATION

MATERIALS
1. Centrifuge
2. Centrifuge tubes
3. Centrifuge tube block
4. Coverglasses
5. Coverglass forceps
6. Filling-pipettes (Wintrobe)
7. Hypodermic needles
8. Methyl alcohol, absolute
9. Microscope and lamp
10. Microslides
11. Pipettes, serologic
12. Slide forceps
13. Stain (Giemsa's)
14. Staining jars (Coplin)
15. Syringes, glass

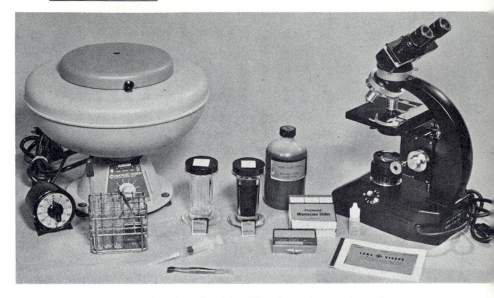

FIG. 2.1.   Materials for the identification of parasites of
the blood.

1. <u>Centrifuge</u>. See Section 1 for specifications.

2. <u>Centrifuge tubes</u>. These are ungraduated, conical tubes of 15
    ml (½ fl oz) capacity. Their length is 12 cm (4¾ in) and the
    diameter is 16 mm (⅝ in).

3. <u>Centrifuge tube block</u>. This may be made from a block of
    wood with several holes bored in it, each hole being 17 mm
    (¹¹⁄₁₆ in) in diameter and 5 cm (2 in) in depth.

4. <u>Coverglasses</u>. Standard 22 mm (⅞ in) squares of plastic or glass
    are recommended.

5. <u>Coverglass forceps</u>. This should always be used when applying
    a coverglass to a specimen on a microslide.

6. <u>Filling-pipettes (Wintrobe)</u>. These are the same pipettes used
    to fill Wintrobe blood sedimentation tubes. They may be pur-
    chased complete with rubber bulbs or made from a 20 cm (8

in) length of glass tubing 7 mm (¼ in) in diameter. The middle of the tubing is heated in the flame of a Bunsen gas burner and, when soft, is drawn out to a diameter of about 1 mm. When cooled, the tube is broken into two pipettes, each about 18 cm (7 in) in length. The larger end of each pipette is provided with a bulb from a medicine dropper.

7. Hypodermic needles. These are 1 inch long, 20 gauge.

8. Methyl alcohol, absolute. This is used prior to staining for the fixation of blood films on microslides.

9. Microscope and lamp. See Section 1 for specifications. An oil-immersion objective is necessary for the proper examination of stained blood films.

10. Microslides. Standard 75 x 25 mm (3 x 1 in) glass slides are used. They must be entirely free from any oily material. After being washed in a warm detergent solution and dried with a clean towel or surgical gauze, the slides are immersed in 70% ethyl (or isopropyl) alcohol and again wiped dry just before they are used.

11. Pipettes, serologic. Their capacity is 1 ml.

12. Slide forceps. This is used for the transfer of blood film slides during fixation and staining procedures. A thumb forceps 12-15 cm (5-6 in) in length is suitable.

13. Stain (Giemsa's). This stain for blood films consists of methanol fixation followed by metachromatic stains. The stain may be purchased ready to use in various-sized units. The method is comparatively rapid and economical and produces films in which differential leukocyte counts may also be made if desired.

14. Staining jars (Coplin). Three staining jars are necessary for staining blood films. Each glass jar is about 12 cm (4⅝ in) high and about 6.5 cm (2⅝ in) in diameter at the base. On the inside are slots to hold five microslides in a vertical position. The

jars have plastic screw-caps to prevent evaporation of the contents.

15. Syringes, glass. Two syringes are necessary, one of 10 ml and the other of 5 ml capacity.

PROCEDURES

In addition to the basic methods described here, various other aids may be used in diagnosis or for the identification of parasites of the blood. Such methods include the inoculation of susceptible animals and intradermal sensitivity testing. Also there are several immunologic tests for the detection of antibodies: the complement-fixation test, fluorescein-labeled antibody test, methylene blue dye test, agglutination test, precipitin test, and flocculation test.

Procedure A

Procedure A is a direct examination of whole blood for the detection of nematode larvae. It is the simplest and most rapid of the procedures to be described for microfilariae.

1. Introduce a sterile 1 inch, 20 gauge hypodermic needle into a vein (e.g. the cephalic vein of dogs).

2. Place a drop of blood from the needle in the center of a clean microslide.

3. Using a coverglass forceps, immediately apply a coverglass to the drop of blood.

4. Place the hypodermic needle in water until it can be cleaned, or wash it immediately.

5. Examine the coverglass area under the low magnification (×100) of the microscope. Look for the undulating movements of nematode larvae. In normal blood the cells may be seen to flow beneath the coverglass. This should not be mistaken for the more violent movements of blood cells when parasitic larvae are present. The larvae may retain their motility for as long as 24 hours on the microslide.

In light infections Procedure A may fail to demonstrate larvae. Therefore, for greater accuracy the other procedures are preferred.

Procedure B

Procedure B is an indirect method for examining whole blood for the detection of nematode larvae, using a centrifuge to separate cells and fibrin from the blood serum.

1. Using a 5 ml sterile glass syringe with a 1 inch, 20 gauge sterile needle attached, slowly withdraw 3–5 ml of blood from a vein (e.g. the cephalic vein of dogs).

2. Slowly discharge the blood from the syringe into a 15 ml centrifuge tube. Allow the blood to clot at room temperature.

3. Immediately rinse the blood from the syringe and needle.

4. Using a piece of metal wire or a disposable wooden applicator stick, rapidly break the clot into small pieces.

5. Centrifuge the blood sample at about 2000 rpm for 3 minutes. This forces the blood cells and fibrin to the bottom of the tube. Nematode larvae will be found in greatest concentration between the clot and the supernatant blood serum.

6. Gently place the centrifuge tube in the wooden block.

7. Using a 1 ml pipette, place the forefinger over the upper end. Insert the pipette through the serum until the tip is just above the clot. Remove the forefinger from the pipette, allowing the serum and larvae to enter.

8. Again close the pipette and withdraw it from the tube. Gently expel the contents onto a clean microslide. Immediately apply a coverglass, using coverglass forceps.

9. Immerse the used pipette in water for rinsing later.

10. Examine the coverglass area under the low magnification ($\times 100$) of the microscope, using a relatively low degree of illumination. In the absence of blood cells, the moving microfilariae are easily seen. They may retain their motility for as long as 48 hours on the microslide and in the centrifuge tube.

Procedure C

Procedure C is an indirect method for examining *hemolyzed* blood for the detection of nematode larvae, using a centrifuge to concentrate them.

1. Draw 4 ml of distilled water into a sterile 10 ml glass syringe which has a 1 inch, 20 gauge sterile needle attached.

2. Slowly withdraw into the same syringe 1 ml of blood from a vein (e.g. the cephalic vein of dogs).

3. Discharge the mixture of water and blood into a 15 ml centrifuge tube.

4. Rinse the syringe and needle for cleaning later.

5. Centrifuge the specimen at 2000 rpm for 3 minutes.

6. Place the centrifuged specimen in the wooden block.

7. Slightly compress the bulb of a filling-pipette; insert the pipette into the bottom of the centrifuge tube and release the bulb, thus removing a small quantity of sediment containing microfilariae.

8. Expel the contents of the filling-pipette onto a clean microslide and immediately apply a coverglass, using coverglass forceps.

9. Examine the coverglass area under the low magnification ($\times 100$) of the microscope, using a relatively low degree of illumination. Nematode larvae will be seen to move, but less actively than those seen using Procedures A or B. Hemolyzed erythrocytes ("ghosts") are seen as dimly outlined bodies. The microfilariae may retain their motility for as long as 24 hours on the microslide and in the centrifuge tube (see Figs. 2.13–2.16).

Procedure D

Knott's technique is a concentration method for the detection of microfilariae in blood.
1. Withdraw 1 ml of blood from the animal to be examined.

2. Mix the blood with 9 ml of 2% formalin solution. (A number of tubes containing 2% formalin solution may be made up ahead of time and let stand until needed.)

3. Centrifuge the mixture at 1200 rpm for 5 minutes and discard the supernatant fluid.

4. Place the sediment on a slide and stain with a drop of 1:1000 aqueous methylene blue solution.

5. Examine under low power ($\times 100$) of the microscope. Microfilariae will be fixed in an extended position, with the nuclei stained blue. Hemolyzed erythrocytes ("ghosts") will be present as dimly outlined bodies.

A ready-made kit for the detection of microfilariae in blood by lysis, filtration, and staining is available commercially as Difil-Test Kit (Evsco Pharmaceutical Corp., Oceanside, N.Y.). The kit provides lysing solution, filters, and staining solution sufficient to conduct 50 tests.

Procedure E

Metachromatic blood stains are very useful for identifying blood parasites. Giemsa's is the most useful, although Wright's stain used in preparing blood films for differential counts is often satisfactory.

1. Place a drop of blood on one end of the slide and, using another slide, draw it out into a thin film as shown in Fig. 2.2.

2. Air-dry the film. Do not blow on it! Protect from flies and other insects if it is not to be stained immediately.

3. Fix in absolute methanol 5 minutes.

4. Air-dry.

5. Dilute stock Giemsa stain (Harleco, Inc., 5821 Market St., Philadelphia, Pa.) 1:20 with distilled water and flood the film.

6. Stain for 30 minutes.

7. Wash stain away gently with tap water.

8. Air-dry. Parasites will stain with blue cytoplasm and magenta nuclei.

(References for Section 2 will be found on pages 250–54)

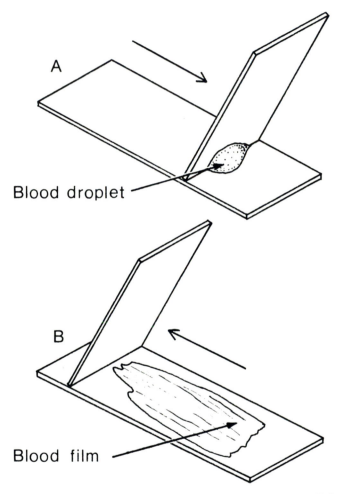

Blood droplet

Blood film

FIG. 2.2.   Technique for making a blood smear: *A*. Bring a spreader slide back at an angle until it touches the drop of blood. Wait until the drop flows laterally. *B*. Draw the spreader slide away from the drop, maintaining an angle. The blood will spread into a smooth, thin film. Practice will result in skill at applying steady, moderate pressure and speed, resulting in uniform films.

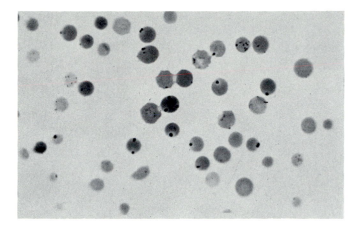

FIG. 2.3.   *Anaplasma marginale* in the erythrocytes of cattle and deer, causing anaplasmosis. This stained blood film was made during the acute febrile stage of the disease, hence the organisms are relatively abundant. × 800.

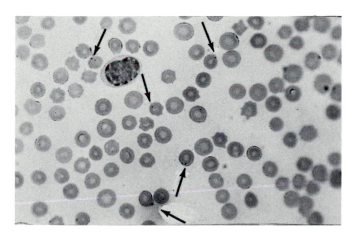

FIG. 2.4.   *Anaplasma marginale.* This stained blood film shows few anaplasms (note arrows). A leukocyte appears at the upper left. × 800.

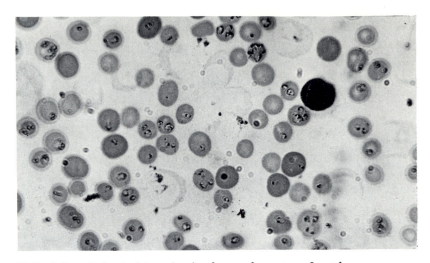

FIG. 2.5. *Babesia bigemina* in the erythrocytes of cattle, the cause of southern cattle fever (babesiasis or piroplasmosis). A leukocyte appears at the upper left. × 800.

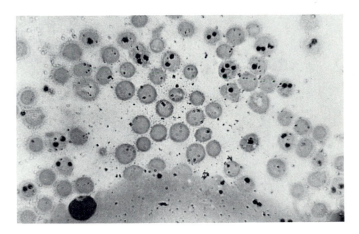

FIG. 2.6. *Babesia canis* in the erythrocytes of dogs, causing canine babesiasis (piroplasmosis). A leukocyte is at the lower left. Numerous artifacts in the form of dust particles appear on the slide. × 800.

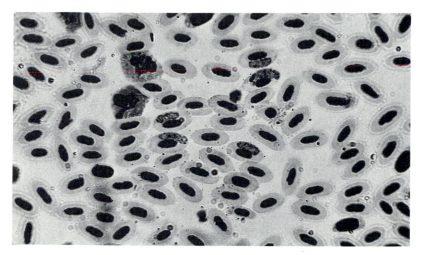

FIG. 2.7. *Haemoproteus columbae,* one of the haemoproteosis organisms causing a malarialike disease of pigeons and doves. The organisms are seen to partially surround the erythrocytic nuclei. Two leukocytes appear at the upper left. × 800.

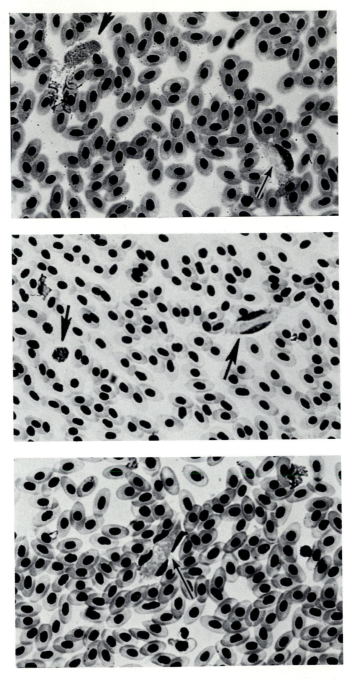

FIG. 2.8. *Leucocytozoon (Leucocytozoon) smithi,* the cause of leucocytozoonosis of turkeys. These three blood films show the protozoa as elongated gametocytes of varying morphology (note arrows). It has not been determined whether these parasites invade leukocytes or erythrocytes or are free in the blood stream. × 600.

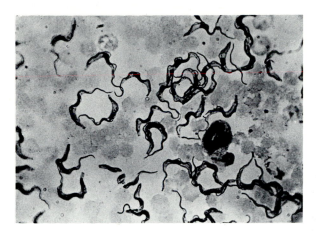

FIG. 2.9. *Trypanosoma equiperdum,* the flagellate protozoon causing dourine in horses. This blood film was taken
from a subinoculated rat. Infected horses show the
trypanosomes more frequently in the genital organs than in
the blood. Dourine is now almost eradicated in North
America. ×1000.

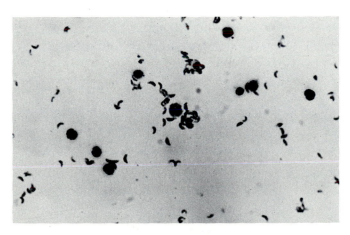

FIG. 2.10. *Toxoplasma gondii,* the cause of toxoplasmosis in many species of mammals, birds, reptiles, and
amphibians. The organism has been found in nearly all
body organs. This smear was made from peritoneal exudate
in a subinoculated mouse. The toxoplasms are the small
crescentic bodies. ×410.

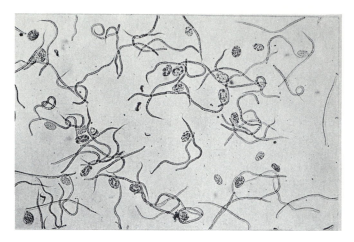

FIG. 2.11.   *Setaria equina* eggs and larvae, obtained by rupturing a female worm from the peritoneal cavity. × 70.

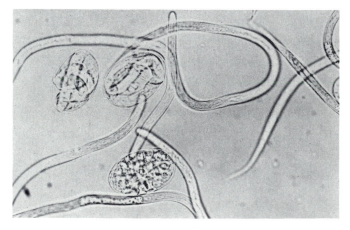

FIG. 2.12.   *Setaria equina* eggs and larvae. × 410.

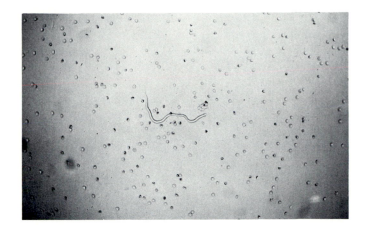

FIG. 2.13.   *Dirofilaria immitis* larva (microfilaria) of the heartworm of dogs, cats, foxes, coyotes, and wolves. This specimen was pipetted from blood serum. × 100.

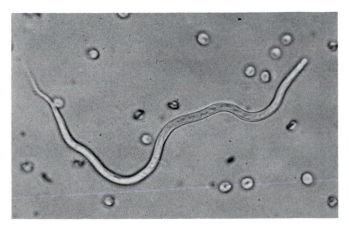

FIG. 2.14.   *Dirofilaria immitis* larva in blood serum. × 410.

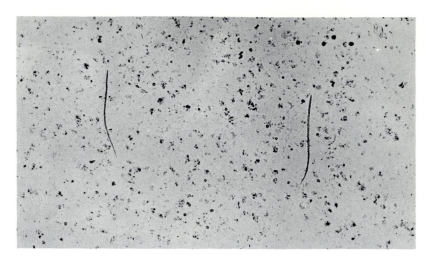

FIG. 2.15.　*Dirofilaria immitis* larvae. The blood sample had been hemolyzed in 2% acetic acid, hence the larvae are almost straight. The outlines of hemolyzed erythrocytes appear in the background. ×100.

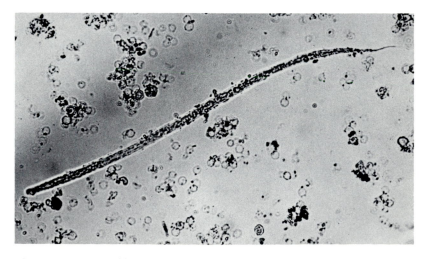

FIG. 2.16.　*Dirofilaria immitis* larva in hemolyzed blood. ×410.

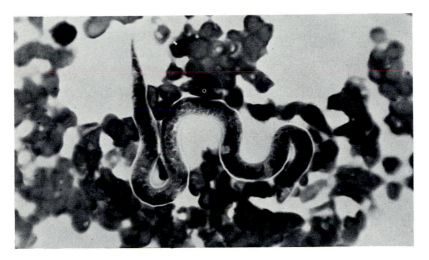

FIG. 2.17.   *Dirofilaria immitis* larva. This specimen is in a
Field's stained whole-blood film. × 800.

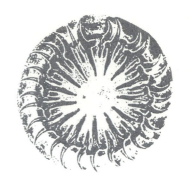

Section Three

MITES AND TICKS (ACARINA)
OF THE SKIN
AND INTERNAL ORGANS

The order Acarina includes the mites and ticks that parasitize domestic animals and man. Mites and ticks belong in the phylum Arthropoda (animals with an exoskeleton and jointed limbs). Arthropods without antennae and mandibles belong in the class Arachnida (spiderlike animals). In the Arachnida is the order Acarina, which includes the mites and ticks; this order comprises arachnids with mouthparts set off from the rest of the body on a false head (capitulum) and in which the body segmentation is greatly reduced or absent.

More than 50 species of mites have been reported to live on or in domesticated mammals and birds of North America. These include the parasitic mange and scab mites, scaly-leg mite, depluming mite, ear mites, feather and quill mites, flesh mite, air-sac mite, chigger mites, roost mite, sinus mite, and nasal mites. For a more complete consideration of parasitic mites (and their control), refer to Baker et al. (1956).

Mites are quite small, most species being either microscopic or under 1 mm in length. They are covered by a relatively soft, often translucent skin through which respiration takes place in the smaller species. The larger species breathe through skin openings (stigmata) connected with tracheal tubes. The body may be ornamented by spines or hairs (setae) or by scalelike plates. The legs (four pairs for adults and nymphs, three pairs for larvae) are provided with clawlike hooks or suctorial cups (see Figs. 3.38, 3.44).

Depending on the species, the food of parasitic mites includes mainly blood, lymph, living and dead epithelial cells, or feathers. Mouthparts are adapted for either piercing or chewing.

The mite life cycle usually begins with the laying of the egg, from which a six-legged larva emerges. After feeding, the skin is shed and the eight-legged but sexually immature nymph appears. Following one or more skin molts, the sexually mature adult mite is formed. Variations occur in the life cycle of certain mite species. For example, the air-sac mite *Cytodites nudus* of poultry is viviparous; the sinus mite *Pneumonyssus caninum* of dogs has not been observed to have a nymph stage.

Ticks are generally larger than mites, being from 4–5 mm long to 12 mm or more in the case of engorged females. Ticks are divided into three families, only two of which are known to be parasitic: the Argasidae (soft ticks) and the Ixodidae (hard ticks). The argasids have a leathery integument, often mammilated and without a dorsal shield or scutum. The life cycle consists of eggs (which are laid in numerous small batches of a few dozen each after a blood meal by the female) and one larval, two nymphal, and one adult stage, with a molt occurring between each stage from larva to adult. The capitulum and mouthparts are ventral and subterminal in the nymphs and adults and thus are not visible from the dorsal view.

The ixodid or hard ticks are so named because of the presence of a hard scutum, which covers the entire dorsal surface of the males but only a small area of the dorsum behind the capitulum in females and immature stages. In some species there may be silvery decorations on the surface of the scutum. The eggs are laid in a single large batch of several hundred to several thousand by engorged females, after which the females die. Posthatch stages include a six-legged larval and eight-legged nymphal and adult stages, with a single molt between each stage. In contrast to the argasids, the mouthparts and capitulum are situated on the anterior margin of the body and are visible from the dorsal aspect.

Ixodid ticks exhibit several life cycle patterns. If the tick remains on the same individual throughout all stages and molts, it is known as a *one-host* tick. In *two-host* species, larva and nymph engorge on the same animal, the nymph drops off and molts, and the adult attacks a new individual. *Three-host* ticks attack a new host after each engorgement, dropping off between stages to molt on the ground.

According to Baker and Wharton (1952), the Acarina are grouped under 4 suborders:

Sarcoptiformes (7 families)
Trombidiformes (5 families)
Mesostigmata (4 families)
Ixodoidea (2 families; see text above)

Following is a brief listing and description of the parasitic mites of domesticated animals by suborders and families.

SUBORDER SARCOPTIFORMES

FAMILY SARCOPTIDAE
Three important genera of mange and scab mites belong in this family: *Sarcoptes, Notoedres,* and *Knemidocoptes.*

Sarcoptic Mange Mites
These mites are the cause of sarcoptic mange or itch. The fertilized females work their way deeply into the epidermis, forming tunnels where they deposit their eggs. Close proximity to nerve endings results in intense irritation. The skin thickens and rather dense crusts form (see Figs. 3.16, 3.17, 3.19, 3.25). The infestation usually involves thin-skinned areas first. There is considerable loss of hair. These mites cause the most common form of mange in swine and horses. The morphologic characteristics of sarcoptic mites are shown in Table 3.1 and Figure 3.1.

TABLE 3.1.   Microscopic Characteristics of the Sarcoptiform Mange and Scab Mites

| Group | Leg Characteristics | | Anus |
	Egg-laying Female	Male	
SARCOPTIC	Sucker on a long *unjointed* stalk on pairs 1 and 2 (Fig. 3.1)	Sucker on a long *unjointed* stalk on pairs 1, 2, and 4 (Fig. 3.1)	Terminal
NOTOEDRIC	As above	As above	Dorsal
KNEMIDO-COPTIC	No suckers (Fig. 3.2)	Sucker on an *unjointed* stalk on pairs 1, 2, 3, and 4 (Fig. 3.2)	Terminal
PSOROPTIC	Sucker on a long *jointed* stalk on pairs 1, 2, and 4 (Fig. 3.3)	Sucker on a long *jointed* stalk on pairs 1, 2, and 3 (Fig. 3.3)	Terminal
CHORIOPTIC	Sucker on a short *unjointed* stalk on pairs 1, 2, and 4 (Fig. 3.4)	Sucker on a short *unjointed* stalk on pairs 1, 2, 3, and 4. Pair 4 rudimentary (Fig. 3.4)	Terminal
OTODECTIC	Sucker on a short *unjointed* stalk on pairs 1 and 2. Pair 4 rudimentary (Fig. 3.5)	Sucker on a short *unjointed* stalk on pairs 1, 2, 3, and 4 (Fig. 3.5)	Terminal

Species and hosts:

Sarcoptes scabiei var. *equi* — horse
Sarcoptes scabiei var. *bovis* — cattle (Figs. 3.16-3.18)
Sarcoptes scabiei var. *ovis* — sheep
Sarcoptes scabiei var. *caprae* — goat
Sarcoptes scabiei var. *suis* — swine (Figs. 3.19-3.24)
Sarcoptes scabiei var. *canis* — dog (Figs. 3.25-3.30)
Sarcoptes scabiei var. *vulpis* — fox

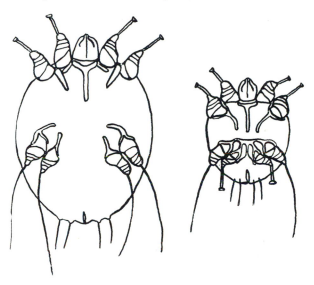

FIG. 3.1.   Female and male mites of the genus *Sarcoptes*, drawn to show the diagnostic features listed in Table 3.1.

Notoedric Mange Mites

These resemble the sarcoptic mites but are somewhat smaller; the anus is located on the dorsal abdominal area rather than terminally (see Fig. 3.32). Notoedric mange is fairly common on cats and rabbits. Lesions are first noticed on the face and other areas of the head, later spreading to various parts of the body, particularly the forelegs. Advanced lesions give cats an appearance of old age because of the wrinkling of the skin of the face. See Table 3.1 for morphology.

Species and hosts:

Notoedres cati — cat, fox (Figs. 3.31-3.34)
Notoedres cati var. *cuniculi* — rabbit

Knemidocoptic Mites

Scaly-leg and depluming scabies of birds are caused by mites of this genus. In the rather common disease scaly-leg, the mites burrow under the scales of the legs and toes, causing dense crusts to form (see Fig. 3.35). Scaly-leg mites are approximately 0.5 mm in diameter and globular in shape. The legs of the adult female are very short; the legs of the male are longer and provided with suckers (see Table 3.1 and Fig. 3.2).

The depluming mite inhabits the skin at the bases of the feathers, especially around the head and neck. Infested birds pick out or scratch out the affected feathers because of the intense irritation. The morphology of depluming mites is much like that of scaly-leg mites, except that the size of the female is approximately 0.35 mm.

Species and hosts:
Knemidocoptes mutans, scaly-leg mite — chicken, turkey, pheasant, caged birds (Figs. 3.36, 3.37)
Knemidocoptes laevis var. *gallinae,* depluming mite — chicken

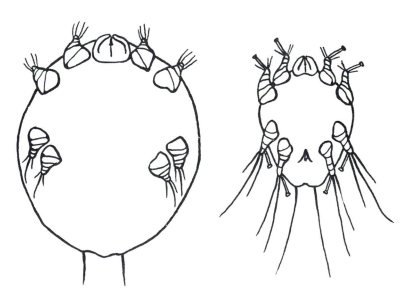

FIG. 3.2. Female and male mites of the genus *Knemidocoptes,* drawn to show the diagnostic features listed in Table 3.1.

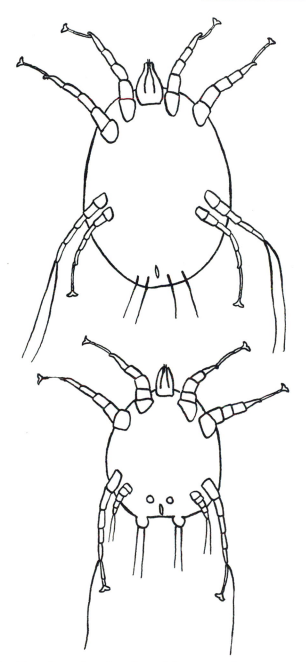

FIG. 3.3.   Female and male mites of the genus *Psoroptes,*
drawn to show the diagnostic features listed in Table 3.1.

FAMILY PSOROPTIDAE

Psoroptic Mites

The mites of this genus are the cause of sheep scab, cattle scab, and similar infestations on other hosts. They differ from the sarcoptic mites in morphology and in their manner of producing lesions. Psoroptic mites do not burrow into the epidermis but remain on the surface or under scabs and scaly accumulations. In addition to the skin of the body, mites of this genus also infest the auditory canals, causing psoroptic ear mange. The lesion is a slight to severe otitis externa, often accompanied by heavy crusting. Sweatman (1958b) revised the mites of the genus *Psoroptes,* reducing the known species to two for domesticated mammals of North America. Psoroptic mites may be as long as 0.8 mm, hence they may be seen grossly or with the aid of a hand magnifier. Magnification of about × 100 is necessary for specific identification (see Table 3.1 and Figs. 3.3, 3.38).

Species and hosts:
Psoroptes ovis—skin of horse, cattle, sheep, and big-horn mountain sheep (Figs. 3.38–3.41)
Psoroptes cuniculi—auditory canals (sometimes body skin) of horse, sheep, goat, and rabbit (Figs. 3.42, 3.43)

Chorioptic Mites

These were formerly known as symbiotic mites. They are the cause of so-called leg, foot, or tail mange. In heavy infestations the abdomen and other parts of the body are involved. The lesions resemble those produced by psoroptic mites; in fact, the mites themselves are quite similar except for the leg details (see Table 3.1 and Figs. 3.4, 3.44) and size. Chorioptic mites reach a maximum length of approximately 0.4 mm. Sweatman (1957) revised the genus.

Species and hosts:
Chorioptes bovis—horse, cattle, sheep, goat (Figs. 3.44–3.48)
Chorioptes texanus—skin of goat, ears of reindeer

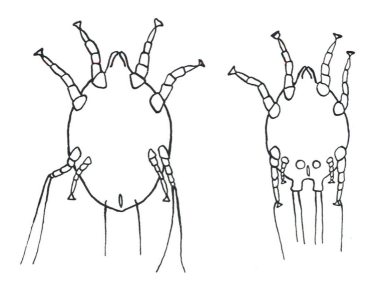

FIG. 3.4. Female and male mites of the genus *Chorioptes*, drawn to show the diagnostic features listed in Table 3.1.

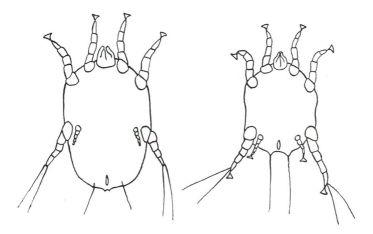

FIG. 3.5. Female and male mites of the genus *Otodectes*, drawn to show the diagnostic features listed in Table 3.1.

Otodectic Mites

As their name implies, these mites invade the ear canals. They are parasites of dogs, cats, foxes, and other carnivora. Their presence is characterized by otitis externa, accompanied by bacterial decomposition of the secretions and the exudate. Ear mites may be seen grossly or with the aid of an otoscope, their size being approximately 0.45 mm in diameter. For specific diagnostic features, see Table 3.1 and Figure 3.5.

Species and hosts:
> *Otodectes cynotis,* ear mite—dog, cat, fox, ferret (Figs. 3.49–3.52)

FAMILY EPIDERMOPTIDAE

This family contains two genera of uncommon skin mites infesting chickens, namely *Epidermoptes* and *Rivoltasia,* each including one species.

Epidermoptes bilobatus causes a rare form of avian scabies which is characterized by brownish yellow elevated scabs on the body and upper portions of the legs. The mites of both sexes have suckers on all of the leg terminations. The length of the adult female is approximately 0.2 mm.

The other species of epidermoptic mite is *Rivoltasia bifurcata,* a feather-eating form, rarely reported from chickens. Apparently only slight damage is done to the infested feathers. These mites are approximately 0.25 mm in length.

Species and hosts:
> *Epidermoptes bilobatus,* scaly-skin mite—chicken
> *Rivoltasia bifurcata,* feather-eating mite—chicken

FAMILY CYTODITIDAE

Cytoditid mites belong to a small group of ectoparasites that have adapted their mode of living to the deeper tissues of the body of the host. The family contains only one species, the air-sac mite of birds.

Cytodites nudus appears to be a fairly common inhabitant of air-sacs, bronchi, lungs, and the bony cavities connected with the respiratory system. It is commonly called the air-sac mite. Hosts include chickens, turkeys, pigeons, and pheasants. Unless air-sac mites are abundant, they apparently do little harm; in large numbers they may be associated with emaciation and anemia. Infected chickens have been known to show symptoms suggestive of avian tuberculosis. Close inspection of the air-sacs soon after the host dies is necessary in order to detect air-sac mites. They may be seen as minute translucent dots, slowly moving about. These mites are less than 0.6 mm in length and resemble the sarcoptic mites.

Species and hosts:
> *Cytodites nudus,* air-sac mite — chicken, turkey, pigeon, pheasant (Figs. 3.56, 3.57)

FAMILY LAMINOSIOPTIDAE

Laminosioptes cysticola is commonly called the subcutaneous mite or flesh mite of birds. Very little is known of its habits. Perhaps it is a skin parasite with a tendency to penetrate to the loose subcutaneous tissues, where it dies. The living mites are seldom observed, probably because they do not produce gross lesions until they die. Most frequently their presence is indicated by yellowish nodules several millimeters in diameter in the subcutis. These nodules appear to be caseocalcareous enclosures around the mites, thus representing a defensive mechanism of the host. Subcutaneous mites are elongated, measuring approximately 0.25 mm long x 0.1 mm wide. A distinctive microscopic feature is the transverse constriction around the body posterior to the second pair of legs.

Species and hosts:
> *Laminosioptes cysticola,* subcutaneous mite — chicken, turkey, goose, pheasant

FAMILY DERMOGLYPHIDAE

These are uncommonly reported inhabitants of the feathers of birds, where they apparently feed, hence the name feather-eating mites.

Falculifer

One species, *Falculifer rostratus,* is a feather-damaging mite of pigeons. It is usually found between the barbs of the large wing feathers, causing the loss of barbules. Its length is approximately 0.5 mm.

Species and host:
> *Falculifer rostratus* — pigeon

Freyana

One subgenus, *Freyana (Microspalax)*, contains the species *Freyana (Microspalax) chaneyi*, which has been reported from turkeys in Maryland, Texas, and Louisiana.

Species and host:
Freyana (Microspalax) chaneyi — turkey

FAMILY ANALGESIDAE

Megninia

This genus of analgesid feather mites is represented by three species in North American domesticated birds.

Megninia gallinulae has been reported only from Canada, and then rarely. It is associated with loss of scales from the lower portions of the legs of chickens and with a crusty dermatitis in the region of the head.

Megninia cubitalis is a similar mite which has been briefly mentioned as occurring on the feathers of chickens and turkeys in southern United States. It is approximately 0.4 mm in length.

Megninia columbae is approximately 0.3 mm in length and has been reported as occurring on the feathers of the neck and body of pigeons in South Carolina.

Species and hosts:
Megninia gallinulae — chicken
Megninia cubitalis — chicken, turkey
Megninia columbae — pigeon

SUBORDER TROMBIDIFORMES

FAMILY DEMODICIDAE

These mites are the cause of demodectic, follicular, or red mange in a variety of hosts. The mites have a distinct appearance. The nonhairy body is elongated; the very short four pairs of legs are situated anteriorly; and the abdomen is transversely striated (see Figs. 3.6, 3.54, 3.55). The adults are approximately 0.1–0.39 mm in length. Demodectic mites live in the hair follicles, sebaceous glands, and the epidermis, where they reproduce. Loss of hair is usually the first symptom of infestation (see Fig. 3.53), followed by dermal hyperemia and eventually by the formation of pustules. The latter are caused by secondary pyogenic bacterial infection. Since

1941 the demodectic mange mite of the dog has been found not only in the hair follicles, sebaceous glands, and epidermis but also in lymph nodes, spleen, kidneys, urine, intestines, feces, and blood (Koutz 1957). The significance of these findings is not yet apparent.

Unsworth (1946), Gaafar et al. (1958), and Koutz et al. (1960) found demodectic mites in the skin of clinically normal dogs. Koutz reported this from 108 of 204 dogs (52.9%).

Although demodectic mange is quite common in dogs, it may also occur in horses, cattle, sheep, goats, and swine. In these less common hosts the only observable lesions may be the formation of cutaneous nodules, varying in size up to 10 or 15 mm in diameter. These nodules are filled with caseous pus containing an abundance of the mites.

Species and hosts:
> *Demodex equi* — horse
> *Demodex bovis* — cattle
> *Demodex ovis* — sheep
> *Demodex caprae* — goat
> *Demodex phylloides* — swine
> *Demodex canis* — dog (Figs. 3.54, 3.55)

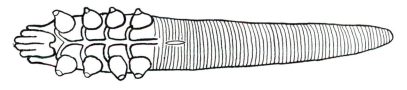

FIG. 3.6.   Female mite of the genus *Demodex,* drawn to show the diagnostic features.

FAMILY TROMBICULIDAE

The trombiculids include the chigger mites, also called redbugs. Only the larval stage is parasitic; the adults and nymphs are free-living or predaceous on insects and other arthropods. Larval chiggers may infest the skin of many mammals, including man, and also the skin of many avian hosts. It is believed their principal hosts are snakes, lizards, turtles, ground birds, and rabbits.

In attacking the host, chiggers insert the mouthparts (chelicerae) and inject a tissue-liquefying saliva. Within a few hours intense pruritus with swelling occurs. The pruritus lasts for days to weeks. Chiggers do not bodily enter the skin while feeding on liquefied tissues. Usually after several hours' attachment they release their hold and drop to the ground for further development. Larval chiggers are difficult to detect on animals. They vary in color from yellowish to red, and their length is about 0.45 mm.

Species and hosts:

Trombicula alfreddugesi, North American chigger — horse, dog, chicken, turkey, and man; also many species of wild mammals, birds, reptiles, and amphibians (Fig. 3.58)

Trombicula batatas — horse, cattle, dog, chicken, turkey, and man; also numerous wild mammals and birds

Trombicula lipovskyana — dog and numerous wild mammals, birds, reptiles, and amphibians

Acomatacarus galli — chicken, mouse, rabbit, rat

Neoschongastia americana, chicken chigger — chicken, turkey, rabbit, and several species of wild birds

FAMILY MYOBIIDAE

Syringophilus bipectinatus, a quill mite, is an inhabitant of the quills of domesticated and wild birds. Its presence is indicated by a powdery accumulation inside the quills of the larger feathers, causing their partial to complete loss. The adult female measures about 0.9 mm in length by about 0.15 mm in width. It is seldom reported.

Syringophilus columbae, the pigeon quill mite, has rarely been reported. It invades the feather quills. Hollander (1956) suggested that an immature stage known as the hypopial nymph is found, often in large numbers, in the connective tissue around the jugular veins and thyroid glands (Fig. 3.59).

Psorergates ovis, the so-called itch mite of sheep, was first reported by Carter (1941) in Australia. Its first occurrence in North America was noted by Bell et al. in Ohio in 1952. Davis (1954) has also studied the sheep itch mite. Infested sheep rub, scratch, or bite at the wool because of a mild chronic dermatitis. Tags of wool hang from the fleece or drop off.

Psorergates mites have legs more or less equidistant apart, whereas the legs of the common mange and scab mites are in groups of two. The adult itch mite of sheep may be as large as 0.189 x 0.162 mm.

Species and hosts:

Syringophilus bipectinatus, quill mite — chicken, turkey, pheasant, other birds

Syringophilus columbae, pigeon quill mite—pigeon
Psorergates ovis, sheep itch mite—sheep

FAMILY CHEYLETIDAE

Cheyletid mites are elongated and possess pincerlike clasping organs (palpi) on each side of the the mouthparts. Most of them are free-living predators of insects or of other mites. *Cheyletiella parasitivorax,* has been reported from the skin of dogs, cats, and rabbits of North America (Cooper 1946; Olsen and Roth 1947; Schaffer et al. 1958). The dog parasite is now considered to be *C. yasguri.*

Cheyletid dermatitis of cats, rabbits, and man has been reported in Europe. Schaffer et al. (1958) reported dermatitis in a bitch and her litter in California. Fleas are known to transport this mite to new hosts. The adult mites are about 0.45 mm long.

Species and hosts:
   Cheyletiella parasitivorax — rabbit
   Cheyletiella yasguri — dog, cat

FAMILY SPELEOGNATHIDAE

A speleognathid mite, *Speleognathus striatus,* was reported in North America from the nasal cavity of the domestic pigeon by Crossley (1952). Its pathogenicity is unknown. Probably it is transmitted through contaminated drinking utensils. The length is about 0.5 mm.

Species and host:
   Speleognathus striatus, nasal mite—pigeon

SUBORDER MESOSTIGMATA

FAMILY DERMANYSSIDAE

Two genera of this family, *Dermanyssus* and *Ornithonyssus,* contain parasites of domesticated birds.

Dermanyssus

One important species, *Dermanyssus gallinae,* is the common chicken mite (red mite, roost mite). Its hosts include chickens, turkeys, pigeons, English sparrows, and other birds. Man and other mammals may be attacked if the mites are abundant. This mite has needlelike mouthparts for sucking blood. Red mites breed in the hosts' surroundings, attacking mostly at night or when the birds are nesting. Adult females, engorged with blood, may reach a length of 1 mm.

Species and hosts:
> *Dermanyssus gallinae,* common red mite — chicken, turkey, pigeon, other birds, occasionally mammals (Fig. 3.60)

Ornithonyssus

Two species of fowl mites have been reported from North America. Although resembling mites of the preceding genus, they differ mainly in that they are found on their bird hosts both day and night, where they suck blood.

The most common fowl mite is *Ornithonyssus sylviarum,* or northern fowl mite. A second species, *Ornithonyssus bursa,* the tropical fowl mite, occurs mainly in the southeastern and south central states. Many birds in addition to chickens are reported to harbor these mites. Adult fowl mites are about 0.8 mm in length.

Species and hosts:
> *Ornithonyssus sylviarum,* northern fowl mite — chicken, man (accidentally), sparrows (Fig. 3.61)
> *Ornithonyssus bursa,* tropical fowl mite — chicken and other bird species

FAMILY RAILLIETIDAE

One species belonging to this family has been rarely reported from cattle in North America. Probably it is more common than the records show. Leidy in 1872 found *Raillietia auris* in the external ear canal of cattle near Philadelphia. It was not until 1950 that it was again reported, this time by Olsen and Bracken in Colorado. Menzies (1957) found this mite in the ear canals of cattle in the vicinity of Austin, Texas. Benbrook (unpublished data) in 1925 identified this mite from the ear canals of a steer that had been shipped into Iowa from Minnesota. This steer showed incoordination and apathy. At necropsy the mites were seen moving rapidly over and near the tympanic membrane. No other evidence was found to account for the symptoms. The adults are approximately 1.5 mm in length.

Species and host:
> *Raillietia auris,* ear mite — cattle (Fig. 3.62)

FAMILY HALARACHNIDAE

The mites of this family occur in the respiratory passages of marine mammals (seals, walruses) and land mammals (carnivores, monkeys, rodents). One species, *Pneumonyssus caninum,* is of interest to veterinarians. This mite occurs quite frequently in the nasal cavity and paranasal sinuses of dogs. Chandler and Ruhe (1940) first described it as a new species. Later references are those of Martin and Deubler (1943), Douglas (1951), Koutz et al. (1953), Furman (1954), Hull (1956), and Besch (1960).

As yet its significance as a pathogen is not clear. Catarrhal or purulent sinusitis may be observed. Mites may be seen crawling from the external nares or slowly moving over the mucosae at necropsy. The mature mites are white and about 2 mm in length.

Species and host:
  Pneumonyssoides caninum, sinus mite — dog (Fig. 3.63)

FAMILY RHINONYSSIDAE

Rhinonyssid mites are parasitic in the nasal passages of various birds. Two species, *Neonyssus columbae* and *Neonyssus melloi,* have been reported in pigeons from Texas by Crossley (1950, 1952). These mites are viviparous, producing larvae in which the nymphs are already developed, according to Baker and Wharton (1952). The adult length is about 0.7 mm.

Species and host:
  Neonyssus columbae, nasal mite — pigeon
  Neonyssus melloi, nasal mite — pigeon

SUBORDER IXODOIDEA

FAMILY ARGASIDAE

Three genera of argasids occur in the United States. Of these only two species, *Argas persicus* and *Otobius megnini,* are commonly parasites of livestock.

Otobius megnini, the spinose ear tick, is a pest of horses and cattle. It is most prevalent in southwestern United States (Fig. 3.64).

Argas persicus, the fowl tick, can be a serious pest of domestic poultry in the Gulf Coast states and southwestern states (Fig. 3.65).

FAMILY IXODIDAE

Seven genera of ixodids, representing at least 13 species of ticks of economic importance as parasites of domestic animals, occur in the United States.

Amblyomma americanum, the Lone Star tick, is generally distributed throughout the southern states from the Rocky Mountains eastward. The tick attacks most domestic animals and man. The common name is derived from the distinctive ornamentation on the scutum of the male (Fig. 3.69).

Amblyomma cajennense, the cayenne tick, is encountered on domestic animals in southern Texas.

Amblyomma maculatum, the Gulf Coast tick, occurs in the Gulf Coast states and attacks numerous domestic animals and man (Fig. 3.70).

Boophilus annulatus, the Texas cattle fever tick, is presently confined south of the Texas-Mexico border. Since this tick is a vector for bovine babesiosis, state and federal authorities should be notified immediately if it is suspected to be present in any area of the United States. Horses, sheep, and goats may be attacked (Fig. 3.67).

Dermacentor albipictus, the winter tick, is distributed in northern and western United States and in Canada. This tick is encountered on the larger domestic animals (cattle and horses) (Fig. 3.71).

Dermacentor andersoni, the Rocky Mountain spotted fever tick, is the woods tick of the western one-third of the United States. It is common on horses, cattle, goats, and man (Fig. 3.73).

Dermacentor nigrolineatus, the brown winter tick, is distributed from the southern plain states into the eastern states. This tick attacks horses, mules, and cattle (Fig. 3.72).

Dermacentor nitens, the tropical horse tick, is found in Texas and Florida. Equine piroplasmosis was apparently introduced into the United States by this tick and is transmitted by it; thus its occurrence should be reported. It is encountered on horses, mules, cattle, and goats.

Dermacentor occidentalis, the Pacific Coast tick, is a parasite of horses, cattle, mules, dogs, and man in Oregon and California.

Dermacentor variabilis, the American dog tick, inhabits brushy areas of the eastern two-thirds of the United States. It is a common parasite of horses, cattle, dogs, and man (Fig. 3.74).

Ixodes scapularis, the black-legged tick, is a parasite of horses, cattle, goats, dogs, and man (Fig. 3.66).

Ixodes pacificus, the California black-legged tick, occurs as a parasite of horses, cattle, dogs, and man in the Pacific Coast states.

Rhipicephalus sanguineus, the brown dog tick, is a cosmopolitan parasite of dogs in the United States. It can become a serious pest in kennel and household situations (Fig. 3.68).

Other ticks may be encountered in the United States. Since many exotic ticks act as vectors of destructive livestock diseases, it is always a sensible procedure to seek expert advice in identification, if any doubt whatsoever exists as to the particular species at hand.

The figures presented are of adult ticks only. Identification of immature stages is more difficult and should be delegated to those skilled in such procedures.

IDENTIFICATION OF PARASITIC MITES

Some species of mites that live on the skin and some of those inhabiting the internal organs may be seen grossly. A hand lens of × 3 or greater magnification is useful for detecting mites if bright lighting is available.

MATERIALS

For the detection and identification of the various microscopic species of mites, it is advisable to take scrapings from the skin or from the internal organs, using the following apparatus:

1. Applicator, cotton-tipped
2. Black paper
3. Coverglasses
4. Coverglass forceps
5. Dissecting needle
6. Hand magnifier
7. Hoyer's solution
8. Jar for waste
9. Medicine dropper
10. Microscope
11. Microscope lamp
12. Microslides
13. Light lubricating oil and dispenser
14. Scalpel
15. Towels or wipes

1. Applicator, cotton-tipped. Wooden applicator sticks 15 cm (6 in) in length are tipped with absorbent cotton. These are for removal of mites from the ear canals.

2. Black paper. Sheets of dull-surfaced black paper about 15 cm (6 in) square are used as backgrounds in the detection of mites, either grossly or with the aid of a hand magnifier.

3. Coverglasses. Any 18 or 22 mm (¾ or ⅞ in) square glass or plastic coverglasses are suitable.

4. Coverglass forceps. This should always be used when applying coverglasses to microslides.

5. Dissecting needle. A wooden- or metal-handled needle is used for picking up individual mites. A stiff sewing needle 5 cm (2 in) long may be set in a 10 cm (4 in) length of 6 mm (¼ in) wooden dowel rod.

6. Hand magnifier. This should provide a magnification of × 3 or more for the examination of mites, ear canal surfaces, or ear swabs. A self-illuminating otoscope may also be used for this purpose.

7. Hoyer's solution. Mites may be permanently fixed in this fluid when mounted on a microslide under a coverglass. For its preparation and use see page 166.

8. Jar for waste. Mites may live for hours after their removal from the host. Discarded swabs, wipes, and slides may be disinfested by placing them in a covered jar containing 3% saponated cresol solution.

9. Medicine dropper. For the transfer of Hoyer's solution to a microslide.

10. Microscope. The same type of microscope and its equipment is recommended as that used for fecal examination (pages 17–19). Lens paper should be used to maintain clean objectives, oculars, condenser, and mirror.

11. Microscope lamp. That used for fecal examination is recommended for mite identification.

12. Microslides. These are standard 75 x 25 mm (3 x 1 in) glass slides. They should be washed and dried before using (if not purchased clean) and may be used repeatedly.

13. Oil and dispenser. Any light-bodied lubricating oil may be used to mount mites temporarily on a microslide under a coverglass. The oil may be dispensed from a small bottle provided with a dropper-pipette, or a small oilcan may be used.

14. Scalpel. A detachable-blade scalpel is preferred for scraping the skin. The blade should be convexly curved.

15. Towels or wipes. Soft woven towels or disposable laboratory wipes are used for drying microslides and for cleaning the scalpel.

TECHNIQUE FOR SKIN EXAMINATION

1. Place a drop of light lubricating oil on a microslide (Fig. 3.7).
2. Clean the scalpel blade by wiping it with paper (Fig. 3.8).
3. Dip the clean scalpel blade into the drop of oil on the microslide (Fig. 3.9).
4. Pick up a fold of the patient's skin at the edge of the suspected area, pinching it firmly between the thumb and forefinger. With the oily scalpel, scrape the crest of the fold several times in the same direction. Scrapings will adhere to the blade. Stop scraping when a slight amount of blood appears (Figs. 3.10, 3.11).
5. Transfer the scraping from the scalpel blade into the drop of oil on the microslide, using a slight rotary motion (Fig. 3.12).
6. Apply a coverglass to the scraping on the microslide by gently lowering it by means of a coverglass forceps. Additional oil may be added at the coverglass edge in order to fill the space beneath it. Do not press on the coverglass (Fig. 3.13).
7. Examine the preparation under low magnification ($\times 100$) in a methodical manner so that all portions of the coverglass area are seen (see Fig. 1.14). For best results, manipulate the substage condenser and diaphragm of the microscope so as to provide a relatively low degree of light evenly distributed.
   Oily preparations of mites may be kept for days as demonstration specimens. The mites show motion for many hours.
8. For the detection of ear mites in the dog, cat, fox, and rabbit, the patient may be restrained in a canvas sheet (Fig. 3.14). A cotton swab is introduced into the external auditory canal and gently rotated. The swab is then placed on a piece of black paper and examined by means of a hand magnifier (Fig. 3.15). Living and dead ear mites may be seen. If necessary, individual

ear mites may be transferred on the tip of the dissecting needle from the cotton swab to a drop of oil on a microslide for microscopic examination. For best results a coverglass should be applied.

An electrically illuminated otoscope cone may be introduced directly into the ear canal for the detection of ear mites, thus making microscopic examination unnecessary.

The more rapidly moving larger skin mites may be captured by touching them with an oily cotton swab. This slows them down so they may be transferred to a drop of oil on a microslide for microscopic examination.

For rapid and permanent mounting of mites, Hoyer's solution may be used:

Distilled water . . . . 50 ml (1.7 fl oz)
Gum arabic flakes . . . . 30 g
Chloral hydrate . . . . 200 g (6.7 oz)
Glycerine . . . . 20 ml

The ingredients are mixed in the order given at room temperature and stored in a tightly sealed container.

Living mites may be directly mounted in this solution. To do this, place a drop of Hoyer's solution on a microslide. Use a dissecting needle to transfer one or more mites to the mounting medium on the slide. Gently lower a coverglass on the specimen, using a coverglass forceps. The slide may then be heated gently in order to hasten the fixing and clearing process.

If mites are to be sent to a diagnostician, they may be immersed in a few ml of 70% ethyl or isopropyl alcohol. Skin scrapings for diagnostic service should be taken from near the edge of an active lesion, avoiding the inclusion of large amounts of dry crusts, hair, or wool. Dried specimens are usually of no value for the identification of mites.

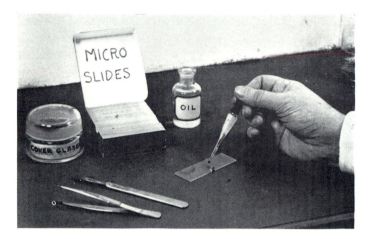

FIG. 3.7. Placing a drop of oil on a microslide.

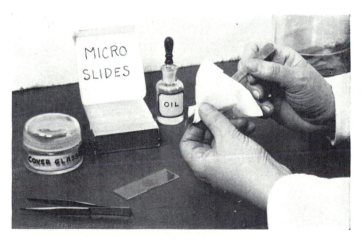

FIG. 3.8. Cleaning the scalpel blade.

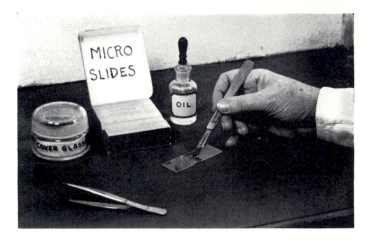

FIG. 3.9. Dipping the cleaned scalpel blade into a drop of oil before scraping the skin.

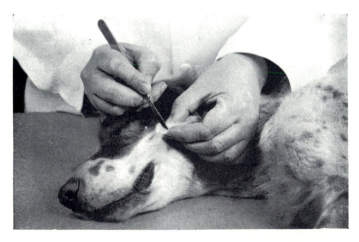

FIG. 3.10. Scraping a fold of a suspected facial lesion with the oiled scalpel blade.

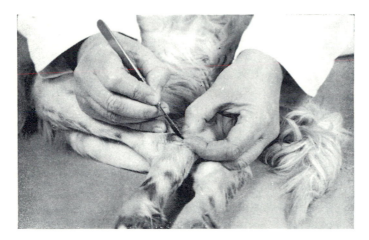

FIG. 3.11.   Scraping a fold of a suspected lesion on the leg.

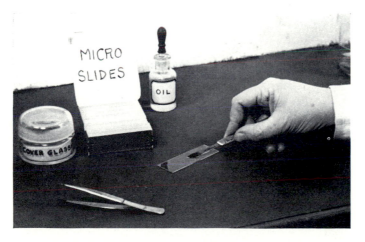

FIG. 3.12.   Transferring the scraping from the scalpel blade to the drop of oil on the microslide.

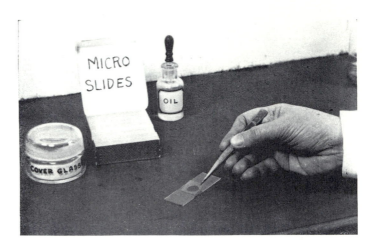

FIG. 3.13.   Applying the coverglass, using forceps.

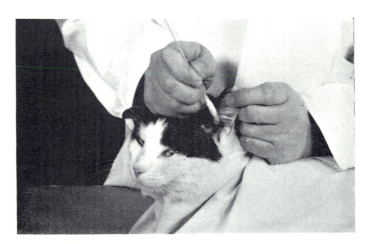

FIG. 3.14.   Removing ear mites on a dry cotton swab. The patient is under restraint in a canvas roll.

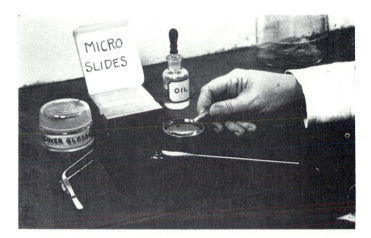

FIG. 3.15. A black paper background and a hand
magnifier are used in examining the cotton swab for ear
mites.

(References for Section 3 will be found on pages 254–57.)

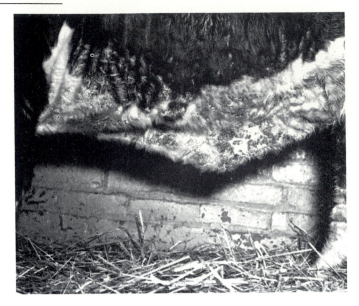

FIG. 3.16. Ventral underline showing encrusted, thickened folds of skin. Lesions caused by *Sarcoptes scabiei* var. *bovis*.

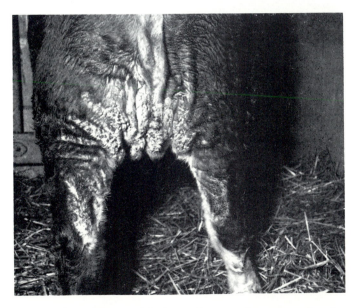

FIG. 3.17. Advanced lesions of sarcoptic mange showing typical encrusted thickened skin thrown up in folds. Lesions caused by *Sarcoptes scabiei* var. *bovis*.

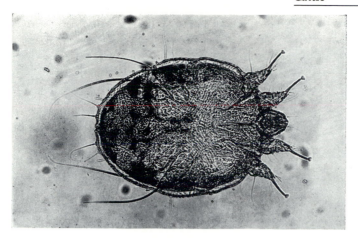

FIG. 3.18.   Adult female *Sarcoptes scabiei* var. *bovis,* the sarcoptic mange mite of cattle. × 130.

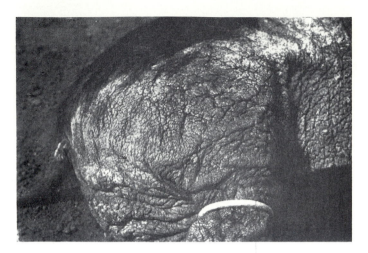

FIG. 3.19. Sarcoptic mange lesion on the hind quarter of a pig.

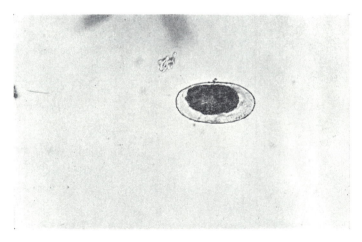

FIG. 3.20. Egg of *Sarcoptes scabiei* var. *suis,* the sarcoptic mange mite of swine. × 100.

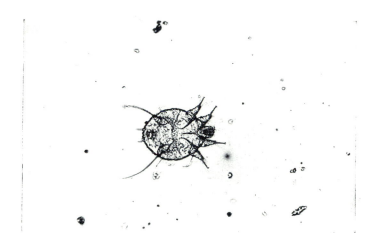

FIG. 3.21.   Larval *Sarcoptes scabiei* var. *suis*. × 100.

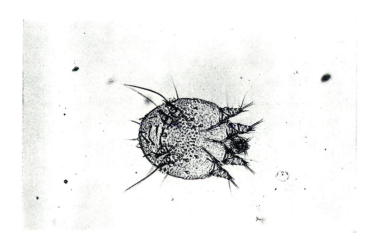

FIG. 3.22.   Nymph of *Sarcoptes scabiei* var. *suis*. × 100.

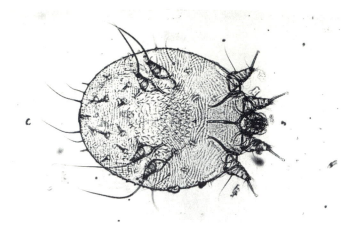

FIG. 3.23.   Adult female *Sarcoptes scabiei* var. *suis.* ×100.

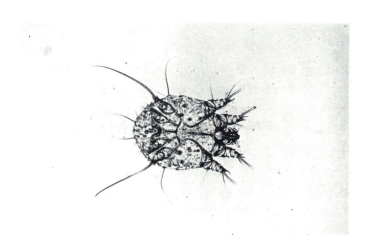

FIG. 3.24.   Adult male *Sarcoptes scabiei* var. *suis.* ×100.

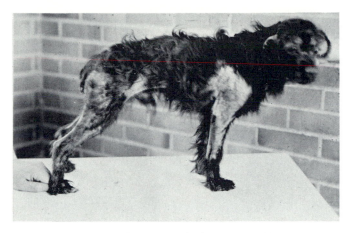

FIG. 3.25.   Sarcoptic mange lesions caused by *Sarcoptes scabiei* var. *canis*.

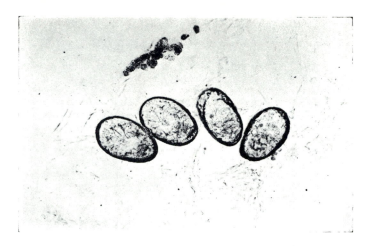

FIG. 3.26.   Eggs of *Sarcoptes scabiei* var. *canis*, the sarcoptic mange mite of dogs. ×100.

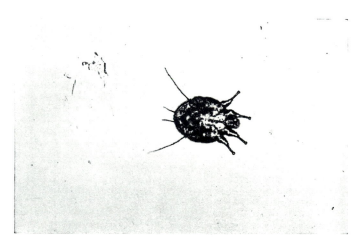

FIG. 3.27.   Larval *Sarcoptes scabiei* var. *canis*. ×100.

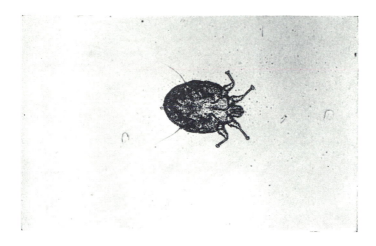

FIG. 3.28.   Nymph of *Sarcoptes scabiei* var. *canis*. ×100.

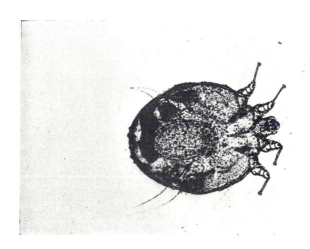

FIG. 3.29.   Adult female *Sarcoptes scabiei* var. *canis*. ×100.

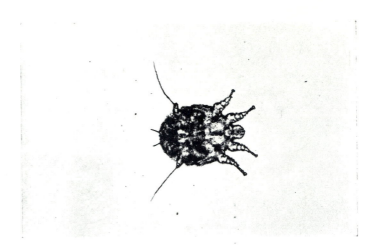

FIG. 3.30. Adult male *Sarcoptes scabiei* var. *canis*. ×100.

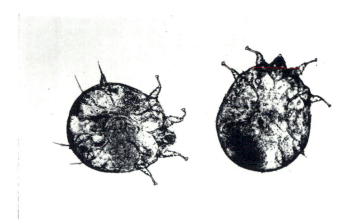

FIG. 3.31. Adult female *Notoedres cati*, the notoedric mange mite of cats, foxes, and rabbits. ×110.

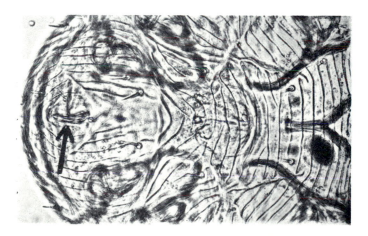

FIG. 3.32. Posterior dorsal abdomen of *Notoedres cati*. Arrow shows the slitlike anus, located dorsally rather than terminally as in the genus *Sarcoptes*. ×410.

FIG. 3.33.   Egg of *Notoedres cati*. × 110.

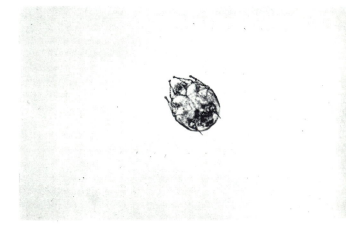

FIG. 3.34.   Larva of *Notoedres cati*. × 110.

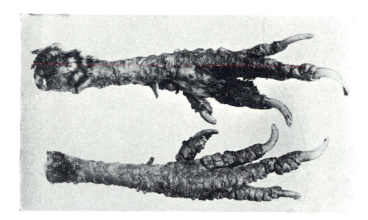

FIG. 3.35. Lesions of scaly-leg on a chicken caused by *Knemidocoptes mutans,* the scaly-leg mite. This or closely related mites cause similar lesions on the lower legs of domesticated turkeys; also pheasants, partridges, and other wild birds. *Knemidocoptes pilae* causes scaly-leg on parakeets.

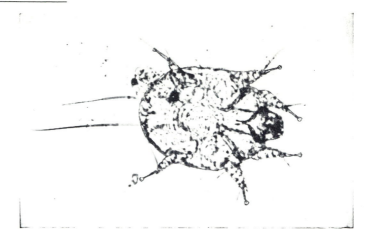

FIG. 3.36.   Larva of *Knemidocoptes mutans,* the scaly-leg mite of chickens, turkeys, and pheasants. ×200.

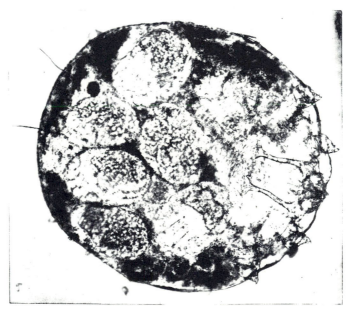

FIG. 3.37.   Adult female *Knemidocoptes mutans.* ×145.

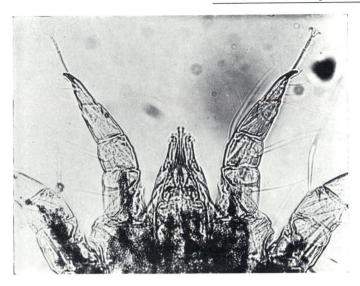

FIG. 3.38.   Details of mouthparts and first pair of legs of *Psoroptes ovis,* the scab mite of horses, cattle, and sheep. The suckers are on long jointed stalks (Table 3.1). ×188.

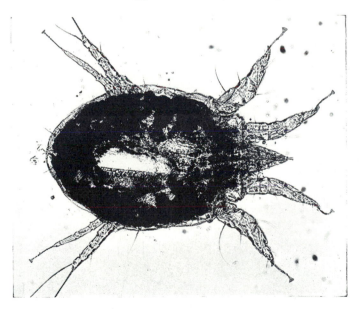

FIG. 3.39.   Egg-laying female *Psoroptes ovis.* ×90.

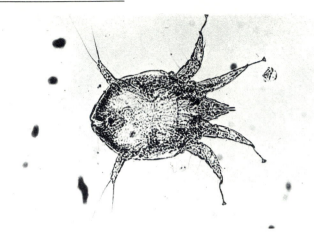

FIG. 3.40.   Larval *Psoroptes ovis*. ×130.

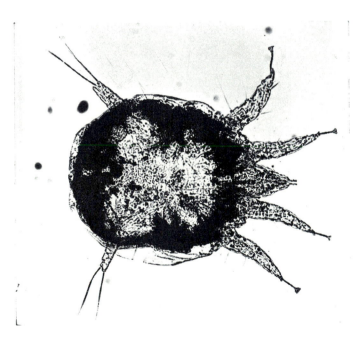

FIG. 3.41.   Pubescent   female   *Psoroptes   ovis*.   The posterior legs (pair 4) are shortened until after copulation. ×120.

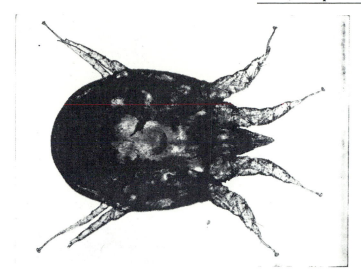

FIG. 3.42. Adult female *Psoroptes cuniculi*, the ear scab mite (sometimes body mite) of horses, sheep, goats, and rabbits. ×75.

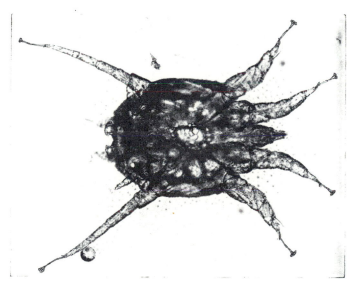

FIG. 3.43. Adult male *Psoroptes cuniculi*. ×75.

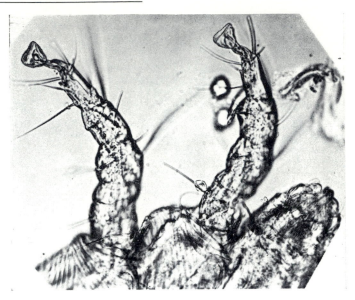

FIG. 3.44.   Details of first and second legs of *Chorioptes bovis*, the chorioptic mange mite of horses, cattle, sheep, and goats. The suckers are on short unjointed stalks (Table 3.1).   ×350.

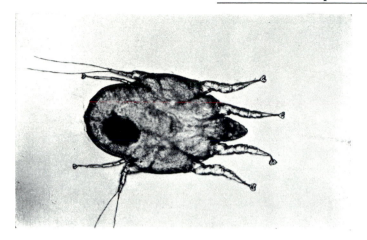

FIG. 3.45.   Adult female *Chorioptes bovis.* × 100.

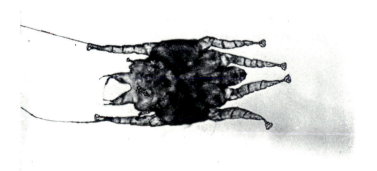

FIG. 3.46.   Adult male *Chorioptes bovis.* × 100.

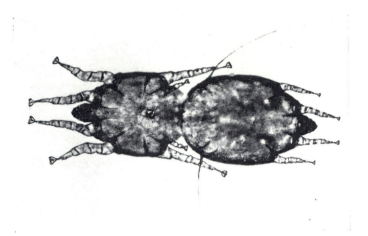

FIG. 3.47.   *Chorioptes bovis* in copulation. × 100.

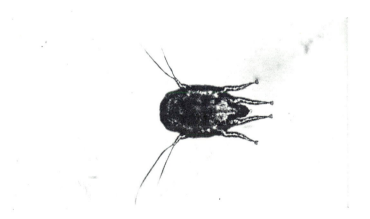

FIG. 3.48.   Larva of *Chorioptes bovis*. Note that there are only three pairs of legs in the larval stage of mites. × 100.

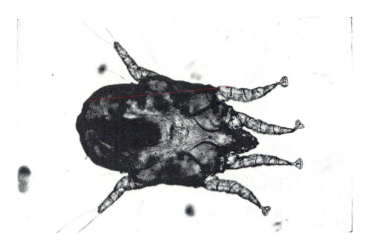

FIG. 3.49.   Adult female *Otodectes cynotis,* the ear mange mite of dogs, foxes, cats, and ferrets. × 100.

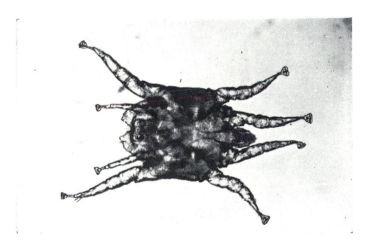

FIG. 3.50.   Adult male *Otodectes cynotis.* × 100.

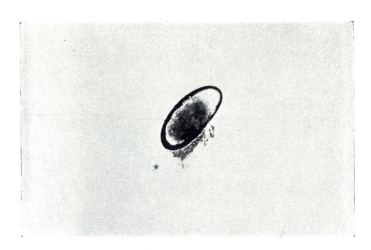

FIG. 3.51.   Egg of *Otodectes cynotis*. × 100.

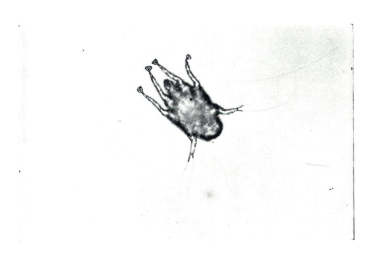

FIG. 3.52.   Larva of *Otodectes cynotis*. × 100.

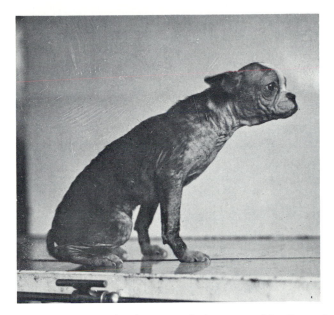

FIG. 3.53.   Demodectic mange lesions caused by *Demodex canis.*

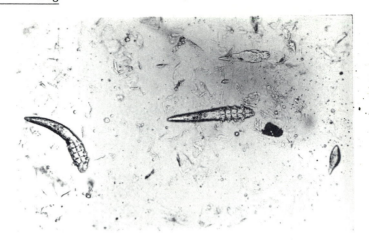

FIG. 3.54.   Adults and an egg *(right)* of *Demodex canis,* the demodectic mange mite of dogs. × 100.

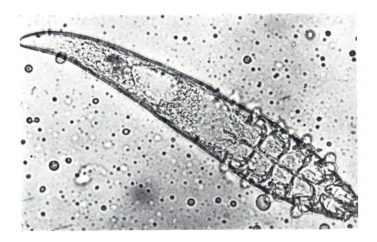

FIG. 3.55.   Adult female *Demodex canis.* × 410.

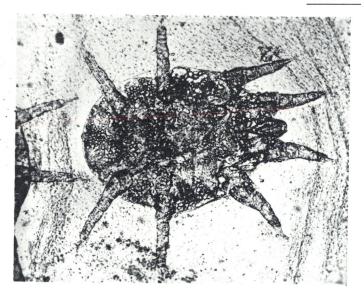

FIG. 3.56.   Adult female *Cytodites nudus,* the air-sac mite of chickens, turkeys, pigeons, and pheasants. A portion of an air-sac appears in the background. ×100.

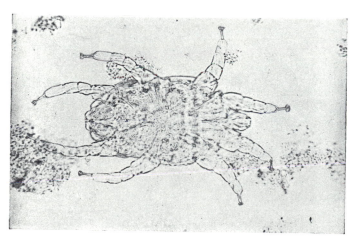

FIG. 3.57.   Adult male *Cytodites nudus.* ×100.

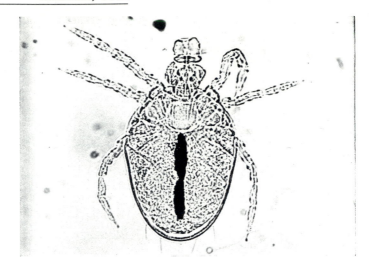

FIG. 3.58.   Larva of *Trombicula alfreddugèsi,* a common chigger mite of horses, dogs, chickens, turkeys, and man; also of many species of wild mammals, birds, reptiles, and amphibians. ×130.

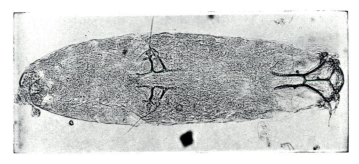

FIG. 3.59.   *Syringophilus columbae,* hypopial nymph stage from connective tissue of a pigeon. The adults are mites inhabiting the feather quills. ×60.

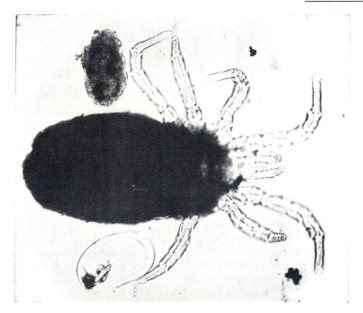

FIG. 3.60. Adult female *Dermanyssus gallinae*, the common red or roost mite of chickens, turkeys, and pigeons; also of man (accidentally), sparrows, and many other wild birds. ×65.

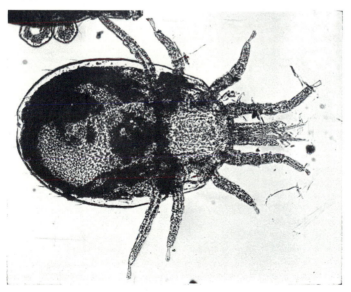

FIG. 3.61. Adult female *Ornithonyssus sylviarum*, the northern fowl mite of chickens; also of man (accidentally), sparrows, and many other wild birds. ×75.

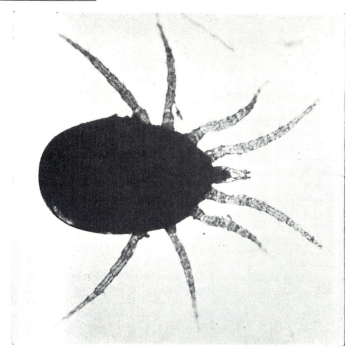

FIG. 3.62.   Adult female *Raillietia auris,* a rarely reported ear mite of cattle. From the tympanic membrane of a steer.

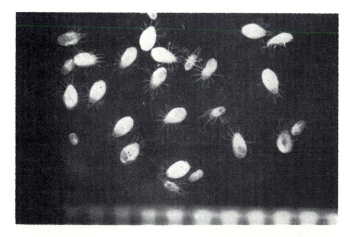

FIG. 3.63.   *Pneumonyssoides caninum,* the frontal sinus mite of dogs. Adults and larvae are seen; also an egg at lower left. Note the millimeter scale below the mites. × 7.

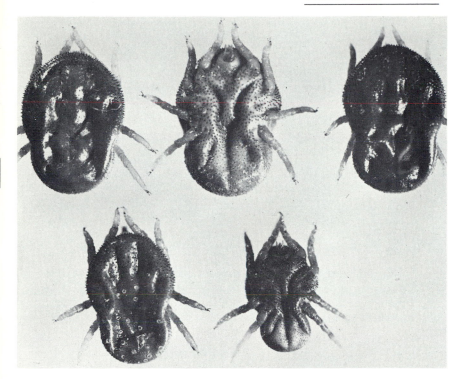

FIG. 3.64.   *Otobius megnini,* the spinose ear tick, nymphal stage II. Most often found in the ears of cattle, dogs,
sheep, and horses; occasionally in goats, pigs, cats, rabbits,
deer, other wild animals, and man. ×6.5.

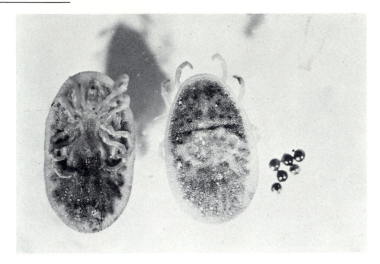

FIG. 3.65. Eggs and dorsal and ventral views of *Argas persicus,* the fowl tick. It attacks fowls, turkeys, pigeons, ducks, geese, canaries, ostriches, and certain wild birds and is known to bite man. × 5.5.

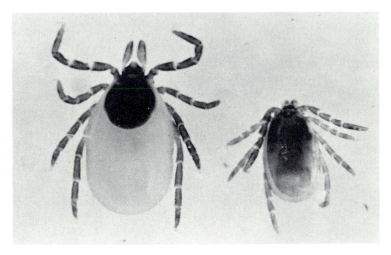

FIG. 3.66. Female *(left)* and male *(right) Ixodes scapularis,* the black-legged tick. The body of the female is usually pale yellow. × 12.

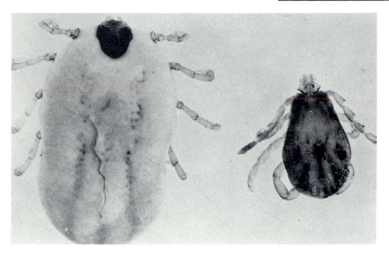

FIG. 3.67. *Boophilus annulatus,* cattle fever tick: *(left)* partially engorged female, *(right)* male. This tick is somewhat similar to *Rhipicephalus sanguineus.* Since it has been eradicated, authorities should be notified if its presence is suspected. × 10.

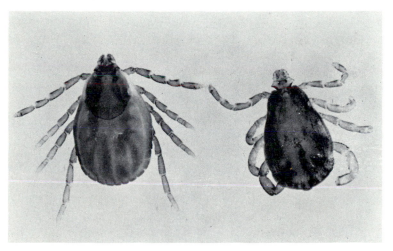

FIG. 3.68. *Rhipicephalus sanguineus,* the brown dog tick: *(left)* engorged female, *(right)* male. This "domesticated" tick is often found crawling in homes. × 10.

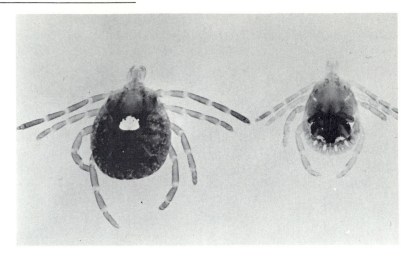

FIG. 3.69. *Amblyomma americanum,* Lone Star tick: *(left)* female, *(right)* male. The single silvery spot on the scutum of the female is characteristic for this tick. ×7.5.

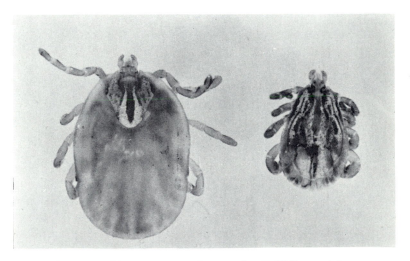

FIG. 3.70. *Amblyomma maculatum,* the Gulf Coast tick: *(left)* partially engorged female, *(right)* male. ×10.

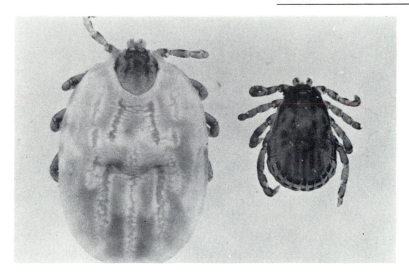

FIG. 3.71. *Dermacentor albipictus,* the winter tick: *(left)* partially engorged female, *(right)* male. ×8.

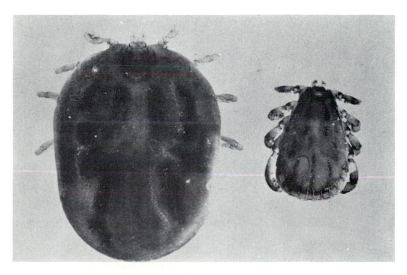

FIG. 3.72. *Dermacentor nigrolineatus,* the brown winter tick: *(left)* engorged female, *(right)* male. ×10.

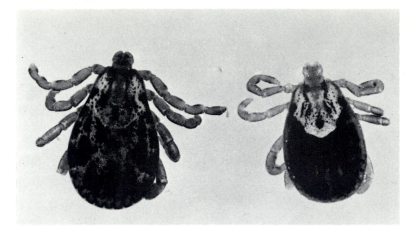

FIG. 3.73. *Dermacentor andersoni,* the Rocky Mountain wood tick: *(left)* male, *(right)* female. The silver coloration of the scutum on the female is usually more complete than on *Dermacentor variabilis.* ×10.

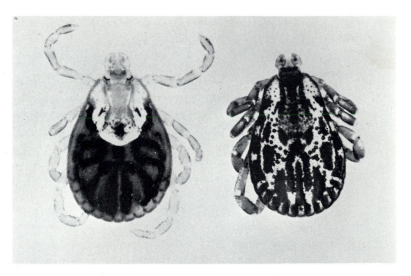

FIG. 3.74. *Dermacentor variabilis,* the American dog tick: *(left)* female, *(right)* male. The silver coloration on the scutum of the female is usually incomplete, forming a U pattern. ×10.

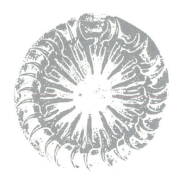

Section Four

LOUSE AND FLEA INFESTATIONS

LICE

Lice are wingless, dorsoventrally flattened insects of the orders Mallophaga or Anoplura, depending on their structure and feeding habits. They are important skin parasites of all domesticated mammals and birds. With few exceptions, each species of lice can live and reproduce on only one host species. The entire life cycle is spent on the host, and transmission is almost entirely by means of host contacts. The length of adult lice varies from slightly more than 1 mm for the smaller species to approximately 5 mm for the larger species. Their bodies are distinctly divided into head, thorax, and abdomen. The three pairs of legs are attached to the thorax. All lice fasten their eggs (nits) to the hair of mammals or to the feathers of their avian hosts. The nymphs that emerge from the eggs are quite similar to the adults except that they are smaller, paler colored, and do not possess mature sexual organs. Most species of lice complete a generation in about three weeks.

DIAGNOSIS

Most lice may easily be seen with the unaided eye. Louse eggs (nits) may likewise be observed, attached to the hair or feathers (see Figs. 4.9, 4.11, 4.12). Bird lice often attach their eggs in clusters at the feather bases (see Fig. 4.22). Chewing lice attract attention by their rapid movements. The examiner may acquire chewing lice on his hands, arms, or body, especially if he handles the cadaver of a louse-infested animal several hours after death.

A hand lens of at least ×3 magnification is very helpful in the detection of lice and their eggs. If microscopic observation is desired, lice may be captured by means of a finely pointed forceps, placed in a drop of water or lubricating oil on a slide, and immobilized by means of a coverglass. Low magnification ($\times 100$) is usually sufficient for the demonstration of morphologic details.

The identification of each louse as to genus and species is beyond the scope of this book. In veterinary diagnosis it is essential that lice be recognized as such; also that the more pathogenic suctorial lice be distinguished from the chewing (biting) species.

MALLOPHAGA

The Mallophaga are the chewing or biting lice, so called because the anteriorly rounded head is provided with mandiblelike mouth parts (see Fig. 4.18). They eat skin scales, feathers, skin secretions, and other organic debris found on the skin. Certain of the bird lice apparently puncture the bases of the young quills, thus obtaining blood. It is quite probable that the biting lice will eat the blood that comes from skin wounds. In general, biting lice are yellow. Their legs are adapted for rapid movement over the skin and its coverings. All species of bird lice and the cat louse are of the biting type. Biting lice also occur on horses, cattle, sheep, goats, and dogs.

Chewing (Biting) Lice of North America

Large Animals

Damalinia equi, biting louse of horses (Fig. 4.1)
Damalinia bovis, red louse of cattle (Fig. 4.3)
Damalinia ovis, biting body louse of sheep (Fig. 4.7)
Damalinia caprae, biting louse of goats, sheep; also dogs (accidentally)
Damalinia limbata, large yellow biting louse of goats
Holokartikos crassipes, biting louse of Angora goats and sheep

Dogs and Cats

Felicola subrostrata, biting louse of cats, bobcats (Fig. 4.16)
Heterodoxus spiniger, biting louse of dogs, coyotes (Fig. 4.14)
Trichodectes canis, biting louse of dogs, coyotes, wolves (Fig. 4.13)

Gallinaceous Fowl

Chelopistes meleagridis, large body louse of turkeys (Fig. 4.21)
Cuclotogaster heterographus, head louse of chickens
Goniocotes gallinae, fluff louse of chickens, guinea fowl (Fig. 4.19)

Goniodes dissimilis, brown louse of chickens, guinea fowl
Goniodes gigas, large body louse of chickens, guinea fowl (Fig. 4.20)
Goniodes numidae, feather louse of guinea fowl
Lipeurus caponis, wing louse of chickens
Menacanthus cornutus, body louse of chickens
Menacanthus pallidulus, small body louse of chickens
Menacanthus stramineus, body louse of chickens, turkeys (Figs. 4.17, 4.18)
Menopon gallinae, shaft louse of chickens, guinea fowl, ducks
Oxylipeurus polytrapezius, slender louse of turkeys

Waterfowl
Anaticola anseris, slender louse of geese
Anaticola crassicornis, slender louse of ducks
Anatoecus dentatus, louse of ducks and geese

Pigeons and Doves
Campanulotes bidentatus, small or golden feather louse of pigeons
Coloceras damnicornis, little feather louse of pigeons
Colpocephalum turbinatum, narrow body louse of pigeons
Columbicola columbae, slender louse of pigeons
Hohorstiella lata, large body louse of pigeons

ANOPLURA

The Anoplura include the suctorial lice. In general they are larger than the chewing lice and are colored gray to dusky red, depending on the amount of host's blood they contain. The head of the suctorial louse is elongated in order to accommodate the protrusible piercing mouthparts. They are comparatively slow moving insects and are most frequently seen head down close to the skin surface. Their legs are adapted for firmly clasping the hair of the host. Suctorial lice are more pathogenic than chewing lice because of their blood-sucking habits. All species of domesticated animals except cats and birds harbor suctorial lice.

Suctorial Lice of North America

Large Animals
Haematopinus asini, sucking louse of horses (Fig. 4.2)
Haematopinus eurysternus, short-nosed louse of cattle (Fig. 4.4)
Haematopinus quadripertussus, tail louse of cattle

Haematopinus suis, common louse of swine (Figs. 4.9–4.12)
Linognathus vituli, long-nosed louse of cattle (Fig. 4.5)
Linognathus ovillus, body and face louse of sheep
Linognathus pedalis, foot louse of sheep (Fig. 4.8)
Linognathus africanus, African blue louse of goats, sheep
Linognathus stenopsis, blue louse of goats
Solenopotes capillatus, little blue louse of cattle, goats (Fig. 4.6)

Small Animals

Linognathus setosus, sucking louse of dogs, foxes, coyotes, ferrets, rabbits, wolves (Fig. 4.15)

FLEAS

Fleas are laterally flattened insects of the order Siphonaptera. Although they are insects, the normal insect division of the body into three parts is not readily apparent. The most characteristic feature is the prominently enlarged third pair of legs which provide the well-known jumping ability. Most fleas are medium to dark brown in color.

Although most important as skin parasites of dogs and cats, fleas of various kinds may occur on any domestic animals or fowls when suitable conditions are allowed to exist. Fleas generally are rather nonspecific in host selection, readily moving to a different host species if a preferred host is unavailable. The life cycle is spent mostly off the host, in the bedding or in the grass; only the adults return to the host temporarily for blood-feeding purposes. As eggs are laid by the females, they fall off into bedding, carpets, grass, or other suitable areas frequented by the host. Adult flea feces in the bedding (see Fig. 4.35) provide feed for the hatched larvae. Pupation occurs after a period of time that varies with temperature and moisture conditions, usually within about two weeks. The adults emerge from the pupal cases fully formed and commence feeding as soon as a suitable host is available.

DIAGNOSIS

Fleas may easily be seen without the aid of magnification. They may be collected most readily by using a rapid-acting insecticidal spray of the pyrethrin type and combing them out of the hair coat of the host. They may be preserved in 70% ethanol in small vials and later mounted in Hoyer's solution (p. 166) on microslides for examination and identification.

Flea identification is a specialized subject and requires considerable expertise for exact speciation. Where this is important, specimens should be submitted to an expert in entomology. The reader should keep this in mind and realize that the photographs provided (Figs. 4.23–4.34) represent only a few of the many possible kinds of fleas encountered.

Each kind may require slightly different control measures, depending on whether they originate primarily from dogs, cats, rats, squirrels, foxes, or other wild animals that may have contact with the environment of the domestic animals.

Fleas of North America

Ctenocephalides canis,   the common dog flea (Figs. 4.23, 4.24). The preferred host is the domestic dog, but wild canids, cats, and man are readily attacked. It serves as the intermediate host for *Dipylidium caninum* (see Figs. 1.106, 1.107).

Ctenocephalides felis, the domestic cat flea, also readily attacks dogs and man. This flea also serves as an intermediate host for *Dipylidium caninum.*

Echidnophaga gallinacea, the tropical hen flea or sticktight flea, also attacks various wild birds and rodents (Figs. 4.25, 4.26).

Nosopsyllus fasciatus, the European rat flea, is found on various rodents, primarily Norwegian and black rats. It can be found on house mice (Figs. 4.29, 4.30).

Orchopeas howardii, the squirrel flea, has also been found on various other wild rodents (Figs. 4.27, 4.28).

Pulex irritans, the human flea, also attacks dogs, cats, swine, and various wild animals (Figs. 4.33, 4.34).

Xenopsylla cheopis, the oriental rat flea, is a dangerous vector of bubonic plague (Figs. 4.31, 4.32).

(References for Section 4 will be found on page 257.)

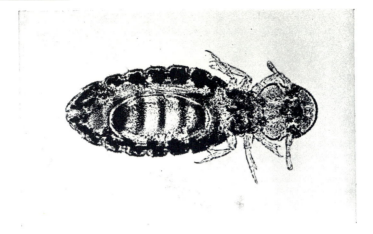

FIG. 4.1.   Adult female *Damalinia equi,* the biting louse of horses. × 32.

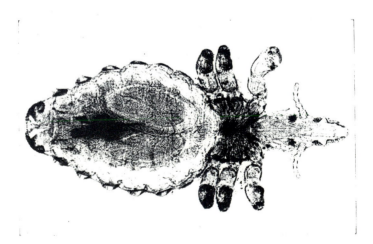

FIG. 4.2.   Adult female *Haematopinus asini,* the suctorial louse of horses. × 25.

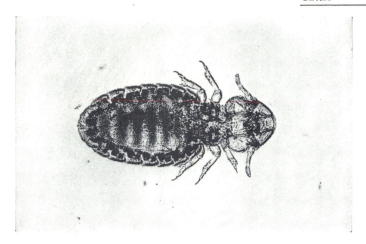

FIG. 4.3.   Adult female *Damalinia bovis,* the biting red louse of cattle. × 32.

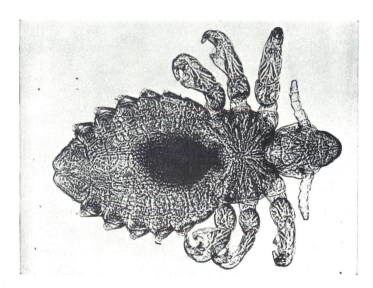

FIG. 4.4.   Adult female *Haematopinus eurysternus,* the short-nosed suctorial louse of cattle. × 40.

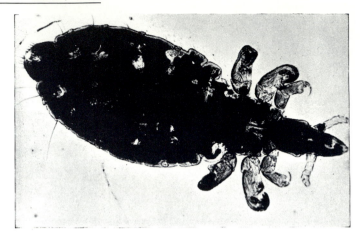

FIG. 4.5. Adult female *Linognathus vituli*, the long-nosed suctorial louse of cattle and goats. ×40.

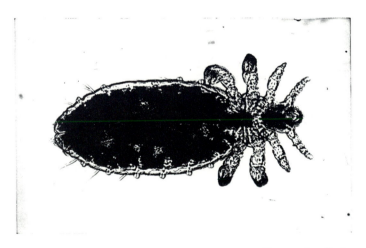

FIG. 4.6. Adult female *Solenopotes capillatus*, the little blue louse of cattle and goats. ×40.

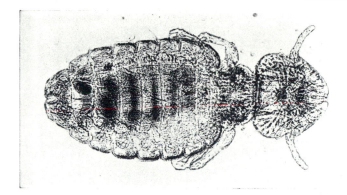

FIG. 4.7. Adult female *Damalinia ovis,* one of the biting lice of sheep. × 50.

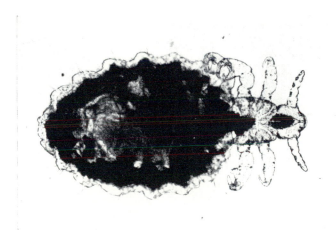

FIG. 4.8. Adult female *Linognathus pedalis,* the suctorial foot louse of sheep. × 37.

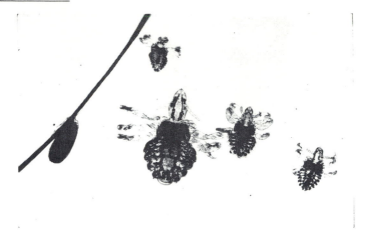

FIG. 4.9. Egg and nymphal stages of *Haematopinus suis,* the swine louse. ×10.

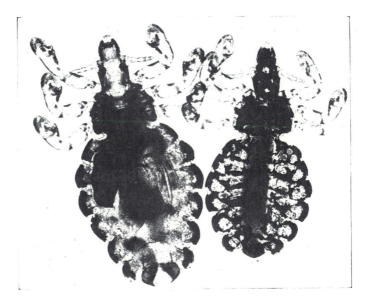

FIG. 4.10. Adult female *(left)* and male *(right)* *Haematopinus suis.* ×15.

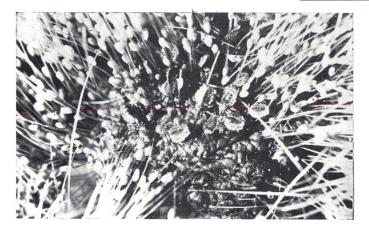

FIG. 4.11.   *Haematopinus suis* and their eggs on the skin.
×1.3.

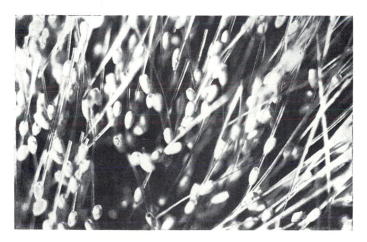

FIG. 4.12.   Eggs of *Haematopinus suis* attached to hairs.
×2.

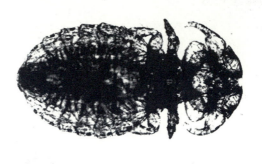

FIG. 4.13.   Adult female *Trichodectes canis,* the common biting louse of dogs and wolves. ×35.

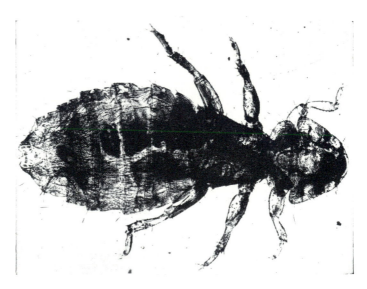

FIG. 4.14.   Adult female *Heterodoxus spiniger,* one of the biting lice of dogs and coyotes. ×40.

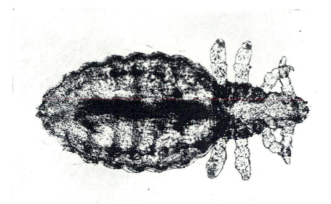

FIG. 4.15. Adult female *Linognathus setosus,* the suctorial louse of dogs and foxes; also of coyotes, ferrets, rabbits, and wolves. ×40.

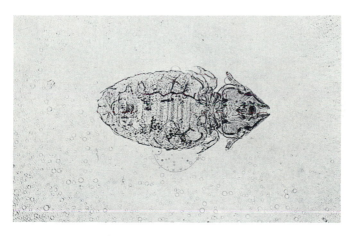

FIG. 4.16. Adult female *Felicola subrostrata,* the biting louse of cats and bobcats. This is the only species of lice found on cats. ×34.

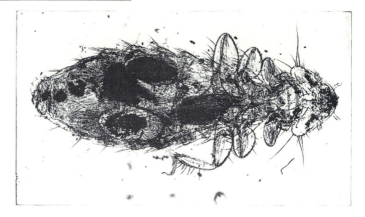

FIG. 4.17. Adult female *Menacanthus stramineus*, the body louse of chickens and turkeys. ×25.

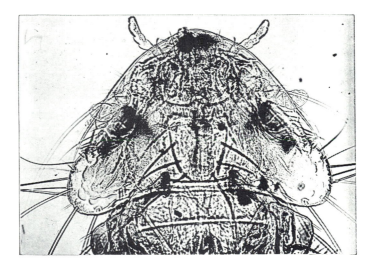

FIG. 4.18. Head of *Menacanthus stramineus*. ×100.

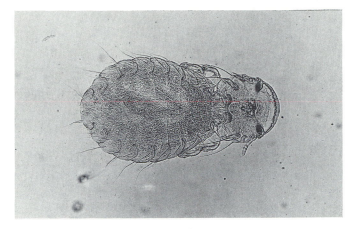

FIG. 4.19.   Adult female *Goniocotes gallinae*, the fluff
louse of chickens and guinea fowl. × 34.

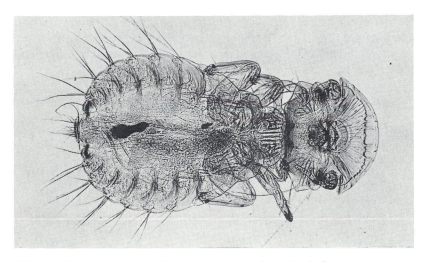

FIG. 4.20.   Adult male *Goniodes gigas*, a large body louse
of chickens and guinea fowl. × 34.

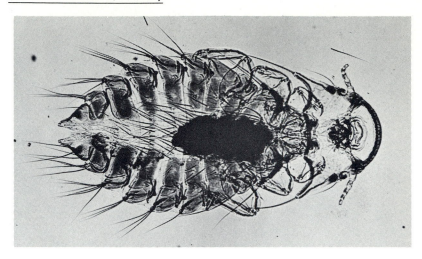

FIG. 4.21. Adult female *Chelopistes meleagridis,* the large body louse of turkeys, both domesticated and wild. ×25.

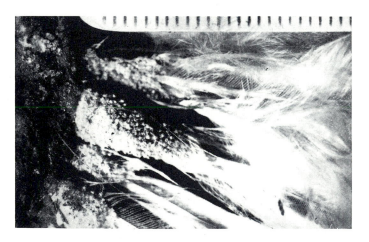

FIG. 4.22. Louse eggs on feather bases of a chicken. ×2.7.

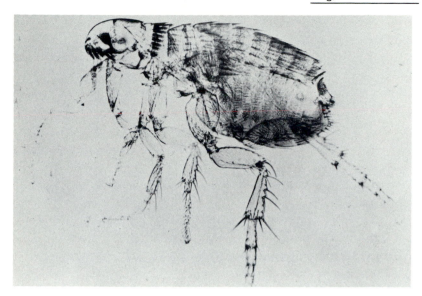

FIG. 4.23. Female *Ctenocephalides canis,* the dog flea. *Ctenocephalides felis* is almost indistinguishable from *C. canis.* Either species may predominate on dogs or cats, depending on the locality. ×30.

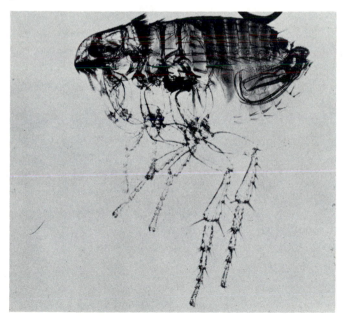

FIG. 4.24. Male *Ctenocephalides canis.* ×30.

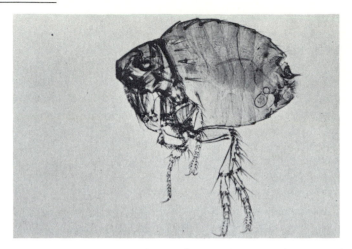

FIG. 4.25.   Female *Echidnophaga gallinacea,* the tropical hen flea or sticktight flea, commonly found on the comb and wattles of fowl. × 40.

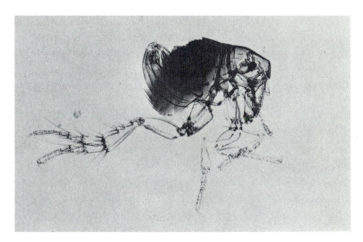

FIG. 4.26.   Male *Echidnophaga gallinacea.* × 40.

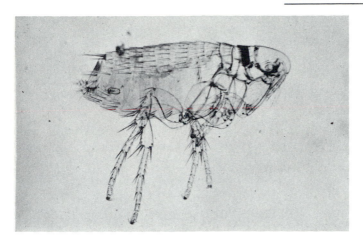

FIG. 4.27. Female *Orchopeas howardii*, the squirrel flea. ×30.

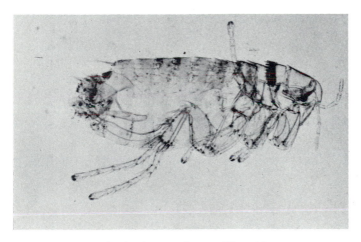

FIG. 4.28. Male *Orchopeas howardii*. ×30.

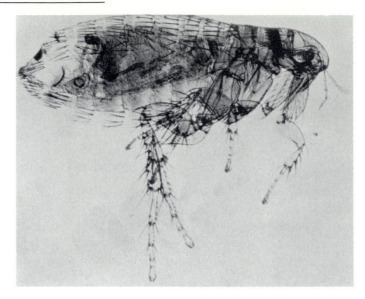

FIG. 4.29.   Female *Nosopsyllus fasciatus,* the rat and rabbit flea. × 40.

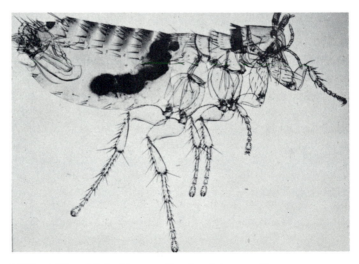

FIG. 4.30.   Male *Nosopsyllus fasciatus.* × 40.

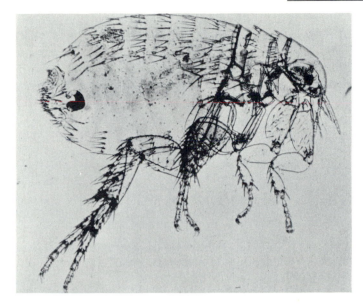

FIG. 4.31. Female *Xenopsylla cheopis,* the plague or rat flea. These fleas of rodents are involved in the transmission of bubonic plague to human beings. ×30.

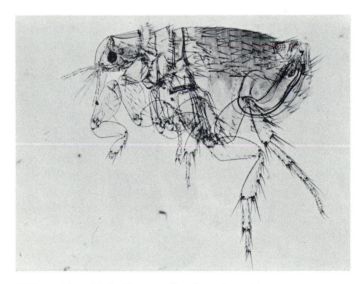

FIG. 4.32. Male *Xenopsylla cheopis.* ×30.

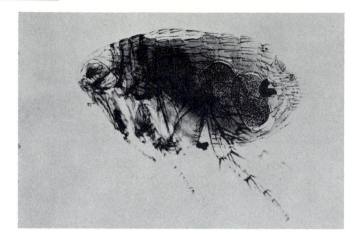

FIG. 4.33. Female *Pulex irritans,* the human flea. Two eggs are visible within the abdomen. × 30.

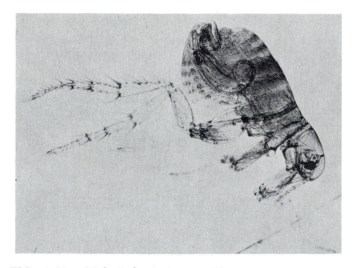

FIG. 4.34. Male *Pulex irritans.* × 30.

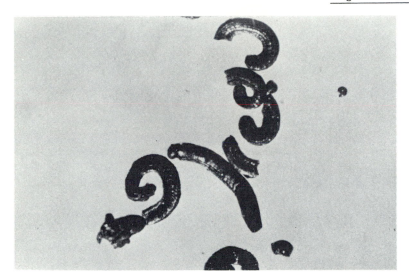

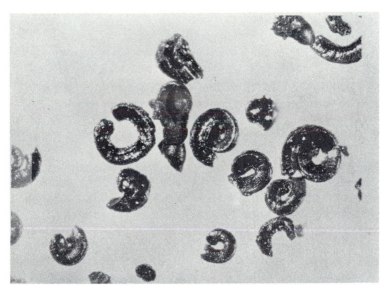

FIG. 4.35.   Flea feces from the bedding of a dog. × 8.

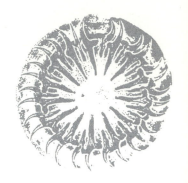

Section Five

MISCELLANEOUS SKIN PARASITES

A number of parasitic or other skin conditions, not convenient-ly discussed in the preceding sections, may be encountered. A few of the more common forms are considered in this section.

FUNGI

In cases of skin disorders not due to nutritional, hormonal, or noninfectious causes, where the presence of mites cannot be substantiated, an examination for the presence of pathogenic fungi should be made. Although identification of fungi is beyond the scope of this manual, some simple techniques and some photographs illustrating typical skin fungi are provided to give the investigator an idea of whether he is dealing with a parasitic or a mycotic condition. It is expected that the reader will consult a more comprehensive source when encountering these conditions.

Many pathogenic fungi will fluoresce with the aid of a Wood's ultraviolet light, but negative results do not preclude the possibility of fungi being present.

A simple method to examine for fungi is to pull some hairs (do not clip) from the periphery of a lesion, defat the hair with ether, and pour off the liquid containing the fat. Soak the hair overnight in a 1% KOH solution. This clears the hair and debris, making spores and hyphae of the fungi visible in or along the hair shafts. A stronger solution of KOH tends to macerate the hair and debris, making the examination difficult (see Figs. 5.1, 5.2).

If time is a factor, another simple method is to pluck the hair and scales from the margin of an active lesion, clear the specimen in

10% KOH by gentle heat, and examine under low magnification with reduced light. Two helpful stains are permanent Black Super Quink Ink (Parker Pen Co.) or the colorant, Ink Blue PP (Fuller Pharmaceutical Co.).

INSECT LARVAE

Callitroga hominivorax, the American screwworm fly, occurs in North and South America, with breeding confined to the southeastern two-thirds of the United States. These flies breed in sores and wounds of numerous host species, including all domestic animals.

Cochliomyia macellaria, the secondary screwworm fly, occurs from southern Canada to southern South America and is a secondary invader of wounds on most domestic animals.

Gasterophilus haemorrhoidalis, Gasterophilus intestinalis, and *Gasterophilus nasalis,* equine stomach bots. The adults deposit eggs on the hairs of the hosts in various locations. These are transferred by licking or by direct skin penetration to the oropharygeal mucosa, eventually migrating to the lumen of the stomach (Figs. 5.3–5.5).

Oestrus ovis, the sheep nose bot. The larvae are deposited around the nostrils and migrate into the nasal cavity and sinuses (Fig. 5.6).

Hypoderma bovis and *Hypoderma lineatum,* the ox warbles or cattle grubs. The eggs are laid on the hairs of the host and eventually reach the subcutaneous tissue of the back after skin penetration and extensive migration occurring over a period of months (Fig. 5.7).

Cuterebra spp., rodent skin bots. The eggs are laid near burrows; the larvae hatch, are swallowed, and migrate to the subcutaneous tissue where cysts are formed. Wild rodents, cats, dogs, and humans are affected (Figs. 5.8, 5.9).

Wohlfahrtia spp., flesh fly. Adult females deposit live larvae in wounds and skin lesions. They are parasites of many animal species (Fig. 5.10).

Sarcophaga spp., flesh fly. Adult females deposit live larvae in wounds and skin lesions. They are parasites of many animal species (Fig. 5.11).

OTHERS

Melophagus ovinus, the sheep ked. Adult females cement larvae, which pupate immediately, to the wool. These are parasites of sheep (Fig. 5.12).

Stephanofilaria stilesi occurs in lesions on the skin of cattle, primarily on the ventral median surface of the abdomen (Figs. 5.13, 5.14).

Cimex lectularius, the bedbug, is a nocturnal insect that hides in crevices and attacks the host for blood meals. It is a parasite of man and poultry (Fig. 5.15).

(References for Section 5 will be found on page 257.)

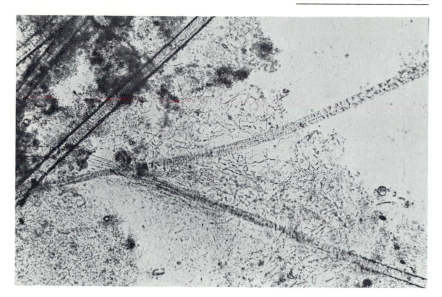

FIG. 5.1. *Trichophyton* spp., a fungus around the hair shaft. ×100.

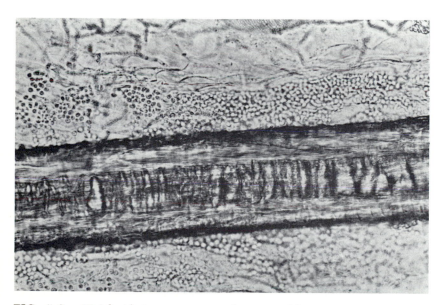

FIG. 5.2. *Trichophyton* spp., a fungus with spores around the hair shafts. ×400.

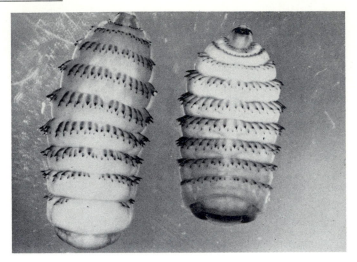

FIG. 5.3. *Gasterophilus intestinalis,* equine stomach bot: *(left)* dorsal, *(right)* ventral. The spines, two rows per segment, are arranged in a staggered pattern, the anterior row consisting of larger spines. ×3.6.

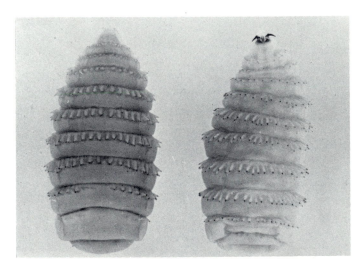

FIG. 5.4. *Gasterophilus nasalis,* equine stomach bot: *(left)* dorsal, *(right)* ventral. The spine pattern is one large row per segment. ×3.75.

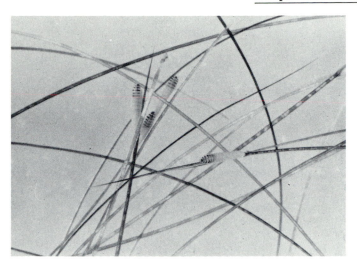

FIG. 5.5. *Gasterophilus intestinalis* eggs. First instar larvae are partially extruded from egg cases attached to distal ends of hairs. ×9.6.

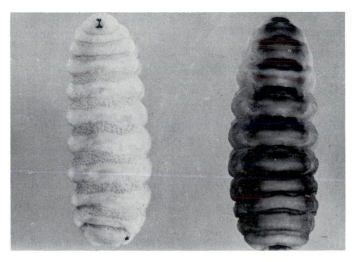

FIG. 5.6. *Oestrus ovis,* sheep nose bot, parasite of nasal cavity and sinuses of sheep and goats: *(left)* ventral, *(right)* dorsal. ×3.

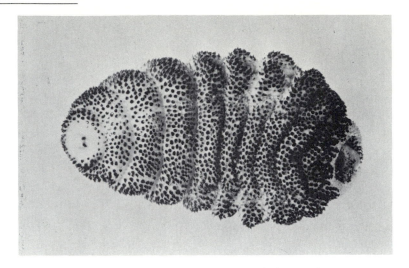

FIG. 5.7. Larva of *Cuterebra* spp., ventral view. × 3.

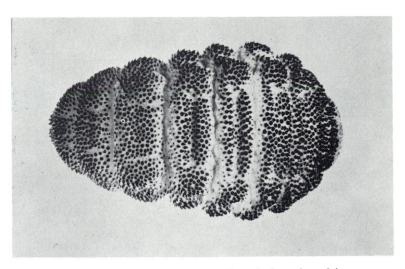

FIG. 5.8. Larva of *Cuterebra* spp., dorsal view, found in the subcutis of a cat. Similar larvae are found in cattle, dogs, sheep, rabbits, mice, and man. × 3.

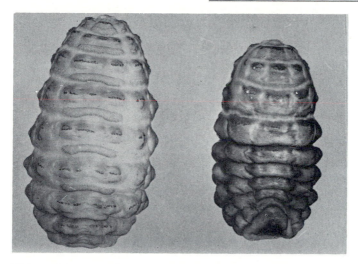

FIG. 5.9. *Hypoderma lineatum,* common cattle grub or ox warble, found in the subcutaneous tissue of the ox: *(left)* dorsal, *(right)* ventral. ×2.7.

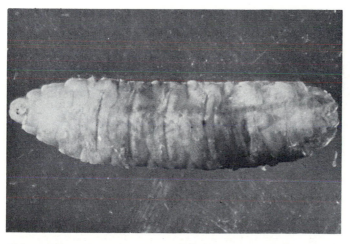

FIG. 5.10. Ventral view of *Wohlfahrtia* sp., flesh fly of various hosts. ×5.1.

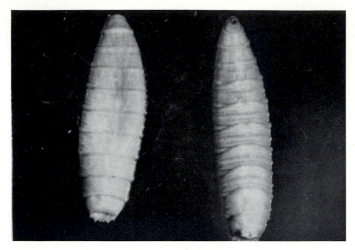

FIG. 5.11. *Sarcophaga bullata*, flesh fly. This and other species infest wounds of various animals: *(left)* dorsal view, *(right)* ventral view. ×2.7.

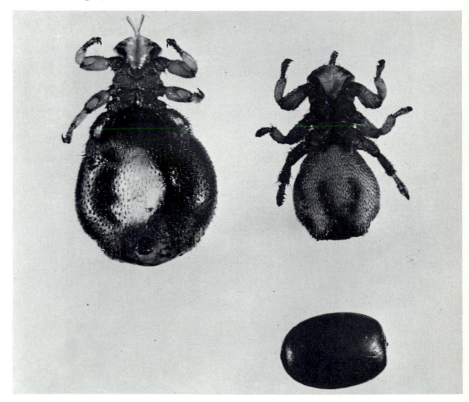

FIG. 5.12. *Melophagus ovinus*, sheep ked (also erroneously called the sheep tick) are found on the skin of sheep: *(left)* female, *(right)* male, *(bottom)* pupa. ×8.

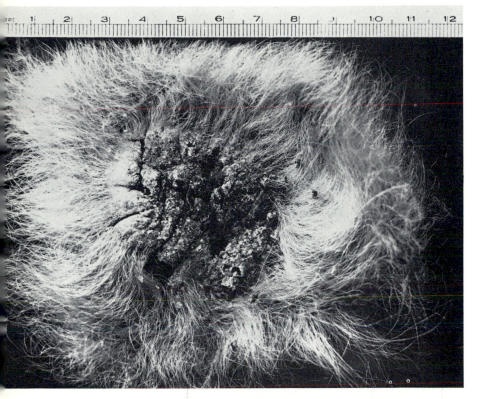

FIG. 5.13.   Lesion caused by *Stephanofilaria stilesi*.

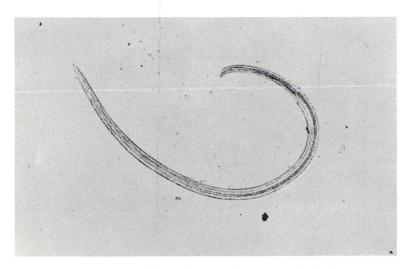

FIG. 5.14.   Male *Stephanofilaria stilesi*, found in lesions on the skin of cattle. ×34.

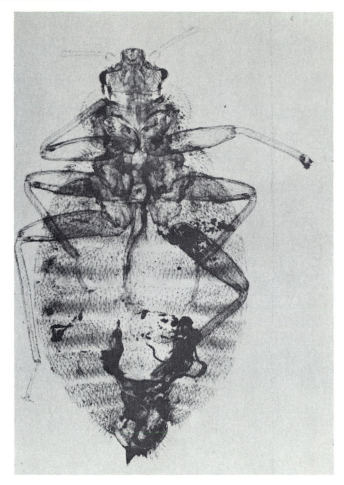

FIG. 5.15.   *Cimex lectularius,* common bedbug. ×20.

REFERENCES

REFERENCES FOR SECTION 1

Alicata, J. E. 1935. (Comparative morphology of eggs and third-stage larvae of some nematodes occurring in swine.) USDA Tech. Bull. 489:85-86.

Anderson, W. R., F. G. Tromba, D. E. Thompson, and P. A. Madden. 1973. Bacteriologic and histologic examination of *Stephanurus dentatus* parasitizing swine ureters. J. Parasitol. 59:765-69.

Ash, L. R. 1970. Diagnostic morphology of the third-stage larvae of *Angiostrongylus cantonensis, Angiostrongylus vasorum, Aelurostrongylus abstrusus,* and *Anafilariides rostratus* (Nematoda: Metastrongyloidea). J. Parasitol. 56:249-53.

Augustine, D. L., M. Nazmi, M. M. Helmy, and E. G. McGavran. 1928. The ovaparasite ratio for *Ancylostoma duodenale* and *Ascaris lumbricoides.* J. Parasitol. 15:45-51.

Bailenger, J. 1959. Coprologie Parasitaire. E. Drouillard, Bordeaux, France.

Bak, I. 1916. Bijdrage tot de diagnostiek der darmparasieten. Ned. Tijdschr. Geneeskd. 60, 2R., 52, pt. 2(13):1117-22.

Bandyopadhyay, A. K., and A. B. Chowdhury. 1961. Autoinfection in strongyloidiasis. Bull. Calcutta Sch. Trop. Med. 9:27.

Baroody, B. J. 1946. Modification of the Faust method in the detection of cysts and ova. J. Lab. Clin. Med. 31:1372-74.

———. 1948. Comparative study of zinc sulfate and saline flotation methods in stool examination. Lab. Diag. 12(2):9.

Barto, L. R. 1936. Fecal analysis of the dog and a study of its importance in clinical diagnosis. North Am. Vet. 17:41-52 (July); 17:39-45 (Aug.).

Bass, C. C. 1910. The diagnosis of hookworm infection, with special reference to the examination of feces for eggs of intestinal parasites. Arch. Diag. 3:231-36.

Bastos, W. D. de A. 1959. Ovos de *Schistosoma mansoni* em fézes de suino *(Sus scrofa)* na Bahia, Brasil. Bol. Inst. Biol. Bahia 4:34-36.

Baughn, C. O., and A. Bliznick. 1954. The incidence of certain helminth parasites of the cat. J. Parasitol. 40(Sec. 2):19.

Bayona-González, A. 1955. Tubo plástico en téchnicas de flotación para investigar parásitos intestinales. Ciencia (Mexico) 14:265-68.

Beach, J. R. 1943. A rapid method for quantitative counts of coccidial oocysts in chicken feces. Cornell Vet. 33:308-10.

Beaver, P. C. 1949a. Quantitative hookworm diagnosis by direct smear. J. Parasitol. 35:125-35.

———. 1949b. A nephelometric method of calibrating the photo-electric light meter for making egg counts by direct fecal smear. J. Parasitol. 35(Sec. 2):13.

———. 1950. The standardization of fecal smears for estimating egg production and worm burden. J. Parasitol. 36:451-56.

Bello, T. R. 1961. Comparison of the floatation of *Metastrongylus* and *Ascaris* eggs in 3 different levitation solutions. Am. J. Vet. Res. 22:597-600.

Benbrook, E. A. 1929. Fecal examination for evidence of parasitism in domestic animals. J. Am. Vet. Med. Assoc. 74(n.s.27):1009-26.

———. 1938. Pine pollen in animal feces. J. Am. Vet. Med. Assoc. 93:46.

Benbrook, E. A., and M. W. Sloss. 1962. Coccidial oocysts *(Eimeria leuckarti)* from North American donkeys *(Asinus asinus).* J. Am. Vet. Med. Assoc. 140:817-18.

Benjamin, M. M. 1961. Outline of Veterinary Clinical Pathology. Iowa State Univ. Press, Ames.

Besch, E. D., R. D. Morrison, and D. L. Weeks. 1960. Preliminary report on the variation in numbers of nematode eggs demonstrated in individual pellets of sheep. Am. J. Vet. Res. 21:917-18.

Biagi, F. F., and J. Portilla. 1957. Comparison of methods for examining stools for parasites. Am. J. Trop. Med. Hyg. 6:906-11.

Blagg, E., E. L. Schloegel, N. S. Mansour, and G. I. Khalaf. 1955. A new concentration technic for the demonstration of protozoa and helminth eggs in feces. Am. J. Trop. Med. Hyg. 4:23-28.

Blount, W. P. 1941. Observations on the modified Gordon-Whitlock method for the counting of helminth ova in horse faeces. J. R. Army Vet. Corps 12:69-78.

Boddie, G. F. 1962. Diagnostic Methods in Veterinary Medicine, 5th ed. J. B. Lippincott, Philadelphia.

Boeck, W. C. 1923. Technique of fecal examination for protozoan infections. Hyg. Lab., U.S. Public Health Serv. Bull. 133:62-74.

Böhm, L. K. 1920. Milben in den Faeces des Hundes; nebst Beiträgen zur Morphologie und Biologie der Milben. Wien. Tieraerztl. Monatsschr. 7:340-46; 361-72.

———. 1928. (Kotuntersuchung auf Parasiten. Tierheilk. u. Tierzucht.) *In:* Stang u. Wirth. Lief. 27, v. 6, pp. 290-304.

Bohrod, M. G. 1945. Detection of *Diphyllobothrium latum* ova in polarized light. Tech. Bull. Regist. Med. Technol. 6:77-78.

Bonilla-Naar, A., and M. Gómez-Vargas. 1948. AEX and "Faust Simplificado" (Bonilla-Naar), two new methods for investigating intestinal parasitism. J. Parasitol. 34(Sec. 2):32 (Abstr.).

Borchert, A. 1959. Morphologische und differentialdiagnostische Angaben über die eklogenen Larvenstadien der Magnefaden-, Knötchen-, Dickdarm- und Zwergfadenwürmer der Schafe. Monatsschr. Veterinaermed. 14:431-37.

Boughton, D. C. 1937. Studies on oocyst production in avian coccidiosis. I. A dilution count technique. Am. J. Hyg. 25:187-202.

Braun, M., and M. Lühe. 1909. Leitfaden zur Untersuchung der Tierischen Parasiten des Menschen und der Haustiere für Studierende Ärzte und Tierärzte. Würzburg.

Britton, J. W. 1937. Studies on the diagnosis of equine strongylidosis, with special reference to fecal and blood examinations. Cornell Vet. 27:290-96.

———. 1938. Rate of egg production of *Strongylus equinus* and *S. vulgaris* as measured by egg counts and qualitative larval cultures. J. Parasitol. 24:517-20.

———. 1938. Studies on the normal variations in the strongyle egg counts of horse feces. Cornell Vet. 28:228-39.

Brown, H. C., and G. E. F. Stammers. 1922. Observations on canine faeces on London pavements: Bacteriological, helminthological and protozoological. Lancet 203(v. 2):1165-67.

Brown, H. W. 1927. A study of the regularity of egg-production of *Ascaris lumbricoides*, *Necator americanus* and *Trichuris trichiura.* J. Parasitol. 14:110-19.

Brown, R. L. 1945. Comparative studies on enterozoic parasite ova and cysts concentrating procedures. Am. J. Trop. Med. 25:375-76.

Brumpt, Emile A. J. 1913. Précis de Parasitologie, 2nd ed. Masson et cie., Paris.

Burch, G. R., and F. A. Ehrenford. 1953. Canine strongyloidiasis. Vet. Med. 48:417-20.

Cabrera, D. J., and W. S. Bailey. 1964. A modified Stoll technique for detecting eggs of *Spirocerca lupi.* J. Am. Vet. Med. Assoc. 145:573-75.

Caldwell, F. C., and E. L. Caldwell. 1926. A dilution-floatation technic for counting hookworm ova in field surveys. Am. J. Hyg. 6 (March suppl.):146-59.

Campori, A. S. 1942. Diagnóstico de las teniasis en el perro por el método del hispo. Univ. Buenos Aires, Rev. Fac. Agron. Vet. 9:170-80.

Castro, G. A., L. R. Johnson, E. M. Copeland, and S. J. Dudrick. 1976. Course of infection with enteric parasites in hosts shifted from enteral to total parenteral nutrition. J. Parasitol. 62:353-59.

Catcott, E. J. 1946. The incidence of intestinal protozoa in the dog. J. Am. Vet. Med. Assoc. 108:34-36.

Caveness, F. E., and H. J. Jensen. 1955. Modification of the centrifugal flotation technique for the isolation and concentration of nematodes and their eggs from soil and plant tissues. Proc. Helminthol. Soc. Wash. 22:87-89.

Cheever, A. W., and K. G. Powers. 1968. Counting of *Schistosoma mansoni* eggs in feces. Comparison of a filtration technique and a dilution technique. J. Parasitol. 54:632-33.

Christensen, J. F. 1938. Species differentiation in the coccidia from the domestic sheep. J. Parasitol. 24:453-67.

──────. 1941. The oocysts of coccidia from domestic cattle in Alabama (U.S.A.), with description of two new species. J. Parasitol. 27:203-20.

Christenson, R. O. 1935. Remarques sur les différences qui existent entre les oeufs de *Capillaria aerophila* et de *Trichuris vulpis*, parasites du renard. Ann. Parasitol. 13:318-21.

Christenson, R. O., and H. H. Earle. 1940. Comparative studies on the morphology of the eggs of nematode worms. J. Ala. Acad. Sci. 12:12.

Christenson, R. O., R. L. Butler, and H. H. Creel. 1942. Studies on the eggs of *Ascaridia galli* and *Heterakis gallinae*. Trans. Am. Microsc. Soc. 61:191-205.

Cobb, N. A. 1904. The sheep fluke. Fluke eggs as a quantitative aid in the diagnosis of the distomiasis of the sheep. Agric. Gaz. N. S. Wales 15:658-69.

Coffin, D. L. 1934. The diagnosis of lungworm disease in domestic ruminants, hogs and foxes by practical office-laboratory procedure. Univ. Pa. Vet. Ext. Quart. 90:41-46.

Courtney, C. H., J. V. Ernst, and G. W. Benz. 1976. Redescription of oocysts of the bovine coccidia *Eimeria bukidnonensis* Tubangui 1931 and *E. wyomingensis* Huizininga and Winger 1942. J. Parasitol. 62:372-76.

Cram, E. B. 1928. Spurious parasites from child and dog. (Banana fibre cells and citrus pulp vesicles.) J. Parasitol. 14:202-3.

Crawley, H. 1921. Observations on the eggs of *Dictyocaulus filaria*. J. Am. Vet. Med. Assoc. 58 (n.s. 11):684-88.

──────. 1925. Eggs of *Ankylostoma caninum*. J. Am. Vet. Med. Assoc. 66 (n.s. 19):487-89.

──────. 1926. Eggs of *Toxascaris limbata*. J. Am. Vet. Med. Assoc. 69 (n.s. 22):493-97.

Crofton, H. D. 1954. Nematode parasite populations in sheep on lowland farms. I. Worm egg counts in ewes. Parasitology 44:465-77.

Crosby, R. G. 1957. Differential diagnosis of nematode ova in cattle. In Threlkeld, W. L. 1958. Some Nematode Parasites of Domestic Animals. W. L. Threlkeld, Blacksburg, Va., pp. 228-35.

Cushnie, G. H., and N. C. White. 1948. Seasonal variation in faeces worm-egg counts of sheep. Vet. Rec. 60:105-7.

D'Antoni, J. S., and V. Odom. 1938. A supplementary basic technique for the recovery of protozoan cysts and helminth eggs in feces. Preliminary communication. U.S. Public Health Serv., Public Health Rep. 53:2202-4.

Deem, A. W., and F. Thorp. 1939. Variation in numbers of coccidia in lambs during the feeding season. Vet. Med. 34:46-47.

Dennis, W. R., W. M. Stone, and L. E. Swanson. 1954. A new laboratory and field diagnostic test for fluke ova in feces. J. Am. Vet. Med. Assoc. 124:47-50.

De Rivas, D. 1928. An efficient and rapid method of concentration for the detection of ova and cysts of intestinal parasites. Am. J. Trop. Med. 8:63-72.

Despommier, D. 1973. A circular thermal migration device for the rapid collection of large numbers of intestinal helminths. J. Parasitol. 59:933-34.

Dewhirst, L. W., and M. F. Hansen. 1961. Methods to differentiate and estimate worm burdens in cattle. Vet. Med. 56:84-89.

Dorney, R. S. 1964. Evaluation of a microquantitative method for counting coccidial oocysts. J. Parasitol. 50:518-22.

Dorsman, W. 1956. A new technique for counting eggs of *Fasciola hepatica* in cattle faeces. J. Helminthol. 30:165-72.

Dubey, J. P. 1975. *Isospora ohioensis* sp. n. proposed for *I. rivolta* of the dog. J. Parasitol. 61:462-65.

──────. 1976. A review of *Sarcocystis* of domestic animals and of other coccidia of cats and dogs. J. Am. Vet. Med. Assoc. 169:1061-78.

Dubey, J. P., and R. H. Streitel. 1976. Further studies on the transmission of *Hammondia hammondi* in cats. J. Parasitol. 62:548-51.

Dubey, J. P., N. Miller, and J. K. Frenkel. 1970. Characterization of the new fecal form of *Toxoplasma gondii* from the feces of cats. J. Parasitol. 56:447-56.

Dubey, J. P., C. V. Swan, and J. K. Frenkel. 1972. A simplified method for isolation of *Toxoplasma gondii* from the feces of cats. J. Parasitol. 58:1005-6.

Ehrenford, F. A. 1953a. Differentiation of the ova of *Ancylostoma caninum* and *Uncinaria stenocephala* in dogs. Am. J. Vet. Res. 14:578-80.

Ehrenford, F. A. 1953b. The incidence of some common canine intestinal parasites. J. Parasitol. 39(Suppl., Sec. 2):34.

———. 1954. Diagnosis of *Physaloptera* in dogs by stool examination. J. Parasitol. 40(Sec. 2):16.

Ehrenford, F. A., R. Napier, and R. W. Eshenour. 1959. Clinical diagnosis of canine whipworm infection. Vet. Med. 54:513-16.

Ehrlich, K. 1927. Eine praktische Methode, Leberegeleier im Kote nachzuweisen. Tieraerztl. Rund. 33:254-55.

Eigenfield, D. D., and C. J. Schlesinger. 1944. An improved flotation method for the recovery of ova from feces. J. Am. Vet. Med. Assoc. 104:26.

Elsdon-Dew, R. 1947. Zinc sulphate flotation of faeces. Trans. R. Soc. Trop. Med. Hyg. 41:213.

Euzéby, J. 1958. Diagnostic Expérimental des Helminthoses Animales. Vigot Frères, Paris.

Eyles, D. E., F. E. Jones, J. R. Jumper, and V. P. Drinnon. 1954. Amebic infections in dogs. J. Parasitol. 40:163-66.

Farr, M. M., and G. W. Luttermoser. 1941. Comparative efficiency of zinc sulphate and sugar solutions for the simultaneous flotation of coccidial oocysts and helminth eggs. J. Parasitol. 27:417-24.

Faust, E. C., J. S. D'Antoni, V. Odom, M. J. Miller, C. Peres, W. Sawitz, L. F. Thomen, J. E. Tobie, and J. H. Walker. 1938. A critical study of clinical laboratory technics for the diagnosis of protozoan cysts and helminth eggs in feces. Am. J. Trop. Med. 18:169-83.

Faust, E. C., W. Sawitz, J. E. Tobie, V. Odom, C. Peres, and D. R. Lincicome. 1939. Comparative efficiency of various technics for the diagnosis of protozoa and helminths in feces. J. Parasitol. 25:241-62.

Fayer, R. 1974. Development of *Sarcocystis fusiformis* in the small intestine of the dog. J. Parasitol. 60:660-65.

Fayer, R., A. J. Johnson, and P. H. Hildebrandt. 1976. Oral infection of mammals with *Sarcocystis fusiformis* bradyzoites from cattle and sporocysts from dogs and coyotes. J. Parasitol. 62:10-14.

Ferguson, F. F., A. Z. de Colon, and M. V. Zayas. 1958. Potassium hydroxide centrifugation method for detection of *Schistosoma mansoni* eggs in feces. J. Parasitol. 44:290.

Fernando, M. A., P. H. G. Stockdale, and S. G. Ogungbade. 1973. Pathogenesis of the lesions caused by *Cyathostoma bronchialis* in the respiratory tract of geese. J. Parasitol. 59:980-86.

Ferriolli, Filho F. 1959. Diagnostico da estrongiloidase. Modifacoes do método de Baermann-Morais. Rev. Inst. Med. Trop. Sao Paulo 1:138-40.

———. 1961a. A new modification of Looss-Baermann's technique for the extraction of larvae of *Strongyloides stercoralis* from stools: The dish technique (trans. title). Rev. Inst. Med. Trop. Sao Paulo 3:9-14 (English summary).

———. 1961b. Studies on the conditions influencing the extraction of larvae of *Strongyloides stercoralis* from stools by the modified Looss-Baermann method: The dish technique (trans. title). Rev. Inst. Med. Trop. Sao Paulo 3:51-60.

Flynn, R. J. 1973. Parasites of Laboratory Animals. Iowa State Univ. Press, Ames.

Foreyt, W. J., and A. C. Todd. 1976a. Development of the large American liver fluke, *Fascioloides magna*, in white-tailed deer, cattle, and sheep. J. Parasitol. 62:26-32.

———. 1976b. Prevalence of coccidia in domestic mink in Wisconsin. J. Parasitol. 62:496.

Foster, W. D. 1912. Analysis of the results of 87 fecal examinations of sheep dogs for evidence of parasitism. Science 35:553-54.

———. 1913. Some atypical forms of the eggs of *Ascaris lumbricoides*. Science (n.s. 37):78.

———. 1914. Observations on the eggs of *Ascaris lumbricoides*. J. Parasitol. 1:31-36.

Frenkel, J. K. 1977. *Besnoitia wallacei* of cats and rodents: With a reclassification of other cyst-forming isosporoid coccidia. J. Parasitol. 63:611-28.

Frenkel, J. K., J. P. Dubey, and N. L. Miller. 1970. *Toxoplasma gondii* in cats: Fecal stages identified as coccidian oocysts. Science 167(3919):893-96.

Fudalewicz-Niemczyk, W. 1962. An essay of determination of threadworm parasitofauna in the digestive tract of sheep on basis of fecal examination (trans. title). Wiad. Parazytol. 8:331-36.

Fudalewicz-Niemczyk, W., and Z. Lenkiewicz. 1960. Variability in egg excretion of stomach and intestine parasites of rams (trans. title). Acta Biol. Cracov. Ser. Zool. 3(2):91-104.

Fülleborn, F. 1920. Die Anreicherungen der Helmintheneier mit Kochsalzlösung. Dtsch. Med. Wochenschr. 46:714-15.

Gates, W. H. 1920. A method of concentration of parasitic eggs in feces. J. Parasitol. 7:49.

Georgi, Jay R. 1974. Parasitology for Veterinarians, 2nd ed. W. B. Saunders, Philadelphia.

Gill, B. S. 1954. Comparative floating efficiency of copper nitrate, common salt, and zinc sulphate solutions as levitating media in a modified Lane's (1923-24) D.F.C. technique for poultry coccidia. Indian J. Vet. Sci. Anim. Husb. 24:249-57.

Goldsby, A. I., and D. F. Eveleth. 1946. The diagnosis of internal parasites of sheep. Vet. Med. 41:398.

Gonzalez, C. J., and M. L. Martos Gutiérrez. 1958. Comparative efficiency of the methods of Watson and Otto, Hewitt and Strahan methods for the concentration of the eggs of *Ascaris lumbricoides* or of *Trichuris trichiura* (trans. title). Rev. Iber. Parasitol. 18:167-79.

Gordon, H. M., and H. V. Whitlock. 1939. A new technic for counting nematode eggs in sheep faeces. J. Counc. Sci. Ind. Res. Aust. 12:50-52.

Goss, L. W., and R. E. Rebrassier. 1922. Demonstration of the examination of the feces of the dog for parasitic infestation. North Am. Vet. 3:177-78.

Graham, Robert, et al. 1939. Microscopic diagnosis of parasitism in domestic animals. Ill. Agric. Exp. Stn. Circ. 496.

Gregoire, C., L. Pouplard, C. Cotteleer, P. Schyns, J. Thomas, and A. Deberdt. 1956. Nouvelle méthode de diagnostic. La distomatose. Ann. Med. Vet. 100:294-303.

Greiner, E. C., G. F. Bennett, M. Laird, and C. M. Herman. 1975. Avian haematozoa. II. Taxonomic keys and color pictorial guide to species of Plasmodium. Wildl. Dis. 68(WD 75-3).

Greve, J. H. 1967. Parasites in domestic animals in Iowa. Iowa State Univ. Vet. 29(2):71-72.

Greve, J. H., E. D. Roberts, and M. W. Sloss. 1964. Paragonimiasis in Iowa. Iowa State Univ. Vet. 26(1):21-28.

Gusev, V. F. 1934. Zur Frage der Coccidien der Einhufer. Arch. Wiss. Prakt. Tierheilkd. 68:67-73.

Habermann, R. T., F. P. Williams, Jr., and W. T. S. Thorp. 1954. Identification of some internal parasites of laboratory animals. U.S. Public Health Serv. Pub. 343.

Haley, A. J. 1954. The use of a surface active agent to facilitate the examination of intestinal contents for helminth parasites. J. Parasitol. 40:482.

Hall, M. C. 1912. A comparative study of methods of examining feces for evidences of parasitism. USDA Bur. Anim. Ind. Bull. 135.

———. 1937. Studies on oxyuriasis. I. Types of anal swabs and scrapers, with a description of an improved type of swab. Am. J. Trop. Med. 17:445-53.

Hall, M. C., and E. B. Cram. 1925. Some laboratory methods for parasitological investigations. J. Agric. Res. 30:773-76.

Harper, K., M. D. Little, and S. R. Damon. 1957. Advantages of the PVA-fixative two-bottle stool collection technic in the detection and identification of intestinal parasites. Public Health Lab. 15:96.

Hausheer, W. C., C. A. Herrick, and A. S. Pearse. 1926. Evaluation of the methods of Stoll and Lane in light hookworm infections, and accuracy in diagnosis of the Willis floatation method. Am. J. Hyg. 6:118-35.

Heidegger, H. 1937. Wurmtafeln zum Bestimmen der wichtigsten Haustierparasiten. Ferdinand Enke, Stuttgart.

Hemmert-Halswick, A. 1943. Infektion mit *Globidium leuckarti* beim Pferd. Z. Veterinaerk. 55:192-99.

Herrick, C. A. 1928. A quantitative study of infections with *Ancylostoma caninum* in dogs. Am. J. Hyg. 8:125-57.

Hill, C. H. 1973. Infectivity of embryonated *Trichuris suis* eggs passed through the digestive tracts of post-weaning pigs. J. Parasitol. 59:580-81.

Hill, C. H., and R. E. Zimmerman. 1954. Use of a standard planetary-type mixing machine for separating eggs of the swine whipworm, *Trichuris suis*, from feces. J. Parasitol. 40(Sec. 2):32.

Hill, C. H., and R. E. Zimmerman. 1957. Further uses of a planetary-type mixing machine adapted for separating worm eggs from feces. J. Parasitol. 43(Sec. 2):31.

Hill, H. C. 1946. Observations on *Ancylostoma* and *Toxocara* infection in experimental and stock dogs. J. Parasitol. 32:210.

Hill, R. B. 1926. The estimation of the number of hookworms harbored, by the use of the dilution egg count method. Am. J. Hyg. 6(July suppl.):19-41.

Hiregaudar, L. S. 1956. A record of *Globidium leuckarti* (Flesch) from a horse in India. Cur. Sci. 25:334-35.

Hobmaier, M. 1922. Globidium-Infektion beim Fohlen. Berl. Munch. Tieraerztl. Wochenschr. 38:100-101.

Hobmaier, M., and P. Taube. 1921. Die Kochsalzmethode bei Untersuchung auf Haustier-parasiten. Berl. Tieraerztl. Wochenschr. 37(44):521-22.

Hunter, G. C., and M. H. Quenouille. 1952. Statistical examination of the worm egg count sampling technique for sheep. J. Helminthol. 26:157-70.

Ishii, Y. 1966. Differential morphology of *Paragonimus kellicotti* in North America. J. Parasitol. 52:920-25.

Jahnes, W. G., and E. P. Hodges. 1947. An improved method of sedimenting *Schistosoma japonicum* and other helminth ova. J. Parasitol. 33:483-86.

James, S. L., and D. G. Colley. 1974. A method for the isolation of *Schistosoma mansoni* eggs. J. Parasitol. 60:1043-44.

Jeska, E. L., and C. J. Gentzkow. 1958. Staining fecal protozoa after fixation in formalin. Am. J. Clin. Pathol. 29:184-85.

Johnson, J. C., Jr., T. B. Stewart, and O. M. Hale. 1975. Differential responses of Duroc, Hampshire, and Crossbred pigs to a superimposed experimental infection with the intestinal threadworm, *Strongyloides ransomi*. J. Parasitol. 61:517-24.

Kates, K. C. 1947. Diagnosis of gastrointestinal nematode parasitism of sheep by differential egg counts. Proc. Helminthol. Soc. Wash. 14:44-53.

Kates, K. C., and D. A. Shorb. 1943. Identification of eggs of nematodes parasitic in domestic sheep. Am. J. Vet. Res. 4:54-60.

Kauzal, G. P., and H. M. Gordon. 1941. A useful mixing apparatus for the preparation of suspensions of faeces for helminthological examinations. Aust. Counc. Sci. Ind. Res. J. 14:304-5.

Keller, A. E. 1934. A comparison of the efficiency of the Stoll egg-counting technique with the simple smear method in the diagnosis of hookworm. Am. J. Hyg. 20:307-16.

Kelly, G. W. 1955. The effect of roughage on the number of eggs of *Haemonchus contortus* per gram of feces from experimentally infected calves. J. Am. Vet. Med. Assoc. 127:449-50.

Kelly, J. D. 1973. Occurrence of *Trichuris serrata* von Linston, 1879 (Nematoda: Trichuridae) in the domestic cat *(Felis catus)* in Australia. J. Parasitol. 59:1145-46.

Kistner, Hyong-Sun Ah, and W. L. Hanson. 1972. Coccidial oocysts from a horse in Georgia. J. Parasitol. 58:709.

Knight, R. A., and H. H. Vegers. 1970. Gastrointestinal nematode parasites from domestic sheep, *Ovis aries*, in Nebraska. J. Parasitol. 56:988-90.

Kofoid, C. A., and M. A. Barber. 1918. Rapid method for detection of ova of intestinal parasites in human stools. J. Am. Med. Assoc. 71:1557-61.

Koutz, F. R. 1941. A comparison of floatation solutions in the detection of parasite ova in feces. Am. J. Vet. Res. 2:95-100.

Koutz, F. R., and R. E. Rebrassier. 1948. Identification and Life Cycles of Parasites Affecting Domestic Animals. Ohio State Univ. Press, Columbus.

Kramer, F. 1925. Vergleichende Untersuchungen über den besten Nachweis von Parasiteneiern im Kot und einige Beobachtungen über die Entwicklung von *Ascaris mystax*. Dtsch. Tieraerztl. Wochenschr. 33:701-3.

Krug, E. S., and R. L. Mayhew. 1946. A comparative study of ova of four species of bovine gastro-intestinal nematodes. J. Parasitol. Suppl.(Sec. 2):17-18.

————. 1949. Studies on bovine gastro-intestinal parasites. XIII. Species diagnosis of nematode infections by egg characteristics. Trans. Am. Microsc. Soc. 68:234-39.

Krull, W. H. 1946. The identification of *Thysanosoma actinioides* infections in sheep by examination of fecal pellets. Trans. Am. Microsc. Soc. 65:351-53.

Kupke, A. 1923. Untersuchungen ueber *Globidium leuckarti* Flesch. Z. Infektionskr. 24:210-23.

Lane, C. 1940. Hookworm diagnosis. Assumptions, alterations, controls, time-lag, rediscoveries: D.C.F. Trans. R. Soc. Trop. Med. Hyg. 33:521-36.

Lapage, G. 1968. Veterinary Parasitology, 2nd ed. Charles C Thomas, Springfield, Ill.

Lapage, G., ed. 1962. Mönnig's Veterinary Helminthology and Entomology, 5th ed. William & Wilkins, Baltimore.

Law, R. G., and A. H. Kennedy. 1932. Parasites of fur-bearing animals. Ontario Dep. Game Fish Bull. 4.

Lee, Keun-Tae, Hong-Ki Min, and Chin-Thack Soh. 1976. Transplacental migration of *Toxocara canis* larvae in experimentally infected mice. J. Parasitol. 62:460-65.

Lee, Y. C., and S. Y. Chung. 1958. Buoyancy test on eggs of swine *Ascaris* and whipworm (trans. title). Mem. Coll. Agric. Natl. Taiwan Univ. 5:15-20.

Lesser, E. 1958. Modification of the formalin-ether fecal concentration technique for use with swine feces. J. Parasitol. 44:318.

Levine, N. D. 1973. Protozoan Parasites of Domestic Animals and of Man, 2nd ed. Burgess, Minneapolis.

———. 1968. Nematode Parasites of Domestic Animals and of Man. Burgess, Minneapolis.

———. 1977. Nomenclature of *Sarcocystis* in the ox and sheep and of fecal coccidia of the dog and cat. J. Parasitol. 63:36–51.

Levine, N. D., and I. J. Aves. 1956. Incidence of gastro-intestinal nematodes in Illinois cattle. J. Am. Vet. Med. Assoc. 129:331–32.

Levine, N. D., and G. R. Campbell. 1971. A check-list of the species of the genus *Haemoproteus* (Apicomplexa, Plasmodiidae). J. Protozool. 18:475–84.

Levine, N. D., and D. T. Clark. 1956. Correction factors for fecal consistency in making nematode egg counts of sheep feces. J. Parasitol. 42:658–59.

Levine, N. D., and V. Ivens. 1965. The Coccidian Parasites (Protozoa, Sporozoa) of Rodents. Illinois Biological Monographs 33. Univ. of Ill. Press, Urbana.

———. 1970. The Coccidian Parasites (Protozoa, Sporozoa) of Ruminants. Illinois Biological Monographs 44. Univ. of Ill. Press, Urbana.

Levine, N. D., K. N. Mehra, D. T. Clark, and I. J. Aves. 1960. Comparison of nematode egg counting techniques for cattle and sheep feces. Am. J. Vet. Res. 21:511–15.

Little, M. D. 1962. Experimental studies on the life cycle of *Strongyloides*. J. Parasitol. 48(Sec. 2):41.

Long, P. L., and J. G. Rowell. 1958. Counting oocysts of chicken coccidia. Lab. Pract. 7:515–18, 534.

Loughlin, E. H., and N. R. Stoll. 1946. An efficient concentration method (AEX) for detecting helminthic ova in feces (modification of the Telemann technic). Am. J. Trop. Med. 26:517–27.

Loveless, R. M., and F. L. Andersen. 1975. Experimental infection of coyotes with *Echinococcus granulosus, Isospora canis,* and *Isospora rivolta.* J. Parasitol. 63:546–47.

Lyons, E. T., and J. H. Drudge. 1975. Occurrence of the eyeworm, *Thelazia lacrymalis,* in horses in Kentucky. J. Parasitol. 61:1122–24.

Lyons, E. T., J. H. Drudge, and S. C. Tolliver. 1973. On the life cycle of *Strongyloides westeri* in the equine. J. Parasitol. 59:780–87.

———. 1976. Studies on the development and chemotherapy of larvae of *Parascaris equorum* (Nematoda: Ascaridoidea) in experimentally and naturally infected foals. J. Parasitol. 62:453–59.

McCorkle, J. K. 1945. Modification of Faust-Meleney technic. Bull. U.S. Med. Dep. 45:420–22.

McDonald, J. D. 1920. Some limitations of the flotation method of fecal examination. J. Lab. Clin. Med. 5:386–91.

McNeil, H. L. 1913. An improved method of extracting ova from stools. J. Am. Med. Assoc. 61:1628.

Madden, P. A., and F. G. Tromba. 1976. Scanning electron microscopy of lip denticles of *Ascaris suum* adults of known ages. J. Parasitol. 62:265–71.

Mahrt, J. 1973. Sarcocystis in dogs and its probable transmission from cattle. J. Parasitol. 59:588–89.

Maldonaldo, J. F. 1956. An evaluation of the standardized direct smear for egg counting in parasitological work. Am. J. Trop. Med. Hyg. 5:888–92.

Maldonaldo, J. F., J. Acosta-Matienzo, and C. J. Thillet. 1953. A comparison of fecal examination procedures in the diagnosis of schistosomiasis mansoni. Exp. Parasitol. 2:294–310.

Maldonaldo, J. F., J. Acosta-Matienzo, and F. Vélez-Herrera. 1954. Comparative value of fecal examination procedures in the diagnosis of helminth infections. Exp. Parasitol. 3:403–16.

Maplestone, P. A. 1924. A critical examination of Stoll's method of counting hookworm eggs in faeces. Ann. Trop. Med. Parasitol. 18:189–94.

———. 1929. A simple method of preserving faeces containing hookworm eggs. Indian J. Med. Res. 16:675–82.

Marquardt, W. C. 1961. Separation of nematode eggs from fecal debris by gradient centrifugation. J. Parasitol. 47:248–50.

Marsh, H. 1936. Observations based on weekly parasite egg counts on feces of lambs and yearling sheep. J. Parasitol. 22:379–85.

———. 1938. Healthy cattle as carriers of coccidia. J. Am. Vet. Med. Assoc. 92(n.s. 45):184–94.

Mayhew, R. L. 1962. Studies on bovine gastrointestinal parasites. XXVI. A flotation method for the recovery of parasitic eggs using cane sugar. Trans. Am. Microsc. Soc. 81:264–67.

Mazzotti, L., and H. Hiranaka. 1957. Aplicacion del metodo de Graham en perros infectados con *Taenia pisiformis*. Rev. Inst. Salubr. Enferm. Trop. 17:29-31.

Mazzotti, L., and M. T. Osorio. 1945. The diagnosis of enterobiasis: Comparative study of the Graham and Hall techniques in the diagnosis of enterobiasis. J. Lab. Clin. Med. 30:1046-48.

Mazzotti, L., D. G. Barranco, and H. Hiranaka. 1957. Use of the analytical balance in the counting of helminth eggs (trans. title). Rev. Inst. Salubr. Enferm. Trop. 17:127-28.

Mello, D. A. 1974. A note on egg production of *Ascaris lumbricoides*. J. Parasitol. 60:380-81.

Melvin, D. M. 1956. Comparison of the direct smear and dilution egg counts in the quantitative determination of hookworm infections. Am. J. Hyg. 64:139-48.

Meyer, M. C., and L. R. Penner. 1958. Laboratory Essentials of Animal Parasitology. W. C. Brown, Dubuque, Iowa.

Milaknis, A. 1953. An improved technic for fecal examination. Vet. Med. 48:41.

Miyazaki, I., and S. Habe. 1976. A newly recognized mode of human infection with the lung fluke, *Paragonimus westermanni* (Kerbert 1878). J. Parasitol. 62:646-48.

Mönnig, H. O. 1928. Dilution egg counting on sheep faeces. Am. J. Hyg. 8:902-9.

Morgan, B. B., and P. A. Hawkins. 1949. Diagnosis of helminth infections. Veterinary Helminthology. Burgess, Minneapolis, pp. 345-64.

————. 1952. Diagnosis of protozoan infections. Veterinary Protozoology. Burgess, Minneapolis, pp. 155-68.

Neilson, J. T. M., and N. D. Nghiem. 1974. The dynamics of *Strongyloides papillosus* primary infections in neonatal and adult rabbits. J. Parasitol. 60:786-89.

Neto, V. M., M. O. A. Corrêa, and G. C. Fleury. 1957. Study of the value of the Rugai, Mattos and Brisola method for identifying nematode larvae in feces (trans. title). Rev. Inst. Adolfo Lutz (Brazil) 17:33-38.

Noble, G. A. 1944. A five-minute method for staining fecal smears. Science 100:37-38. (for protozoa)

Nöller, W., and L. Otten. 1921. Die Kochsalzmethode bei der Untersuchung der Haustierkokzidien. Berl. Tieraerztl. Wochenschr. 37:481-83.

Nöller, W., and F. Schmid. 1927. Die Wasserglas-Zentrifugier-Schwimm-Methode nach Vajda 1927 in ihrem Werte für parasitologische Untersuchungen. Tieraerztl. Rund. 33:759-61.

Obitz, K. 1934. Recherches sur les oeufs de quelques anoplocéphalidés. Ann. Parasitol. 12:40-55.

Otto, G. F., R. Hewitt, and D. E. Strahan. 1941. A simplified zinc sulfate levitation method of fecal examination for protozoan cysts and hookworm eggs. Am. J. Hyg. 33:32-37.

Pérez-Fontana, V. 1954. Investigations on eggs of helminths, with special reference to the epidemiology of hydatid disease. Am. J. Trop. Med. Hyg. 3:762-63.

Pesigan, T. P. 1940. Comparative efficiency of zinc sulphate and cupric nitrate technics for the diagnosis of helminth ova and protozoan cysts in feces. Univ. Philippines Nat. Appl. Sci. Bull. 7:305-17.

Peters, B. G., and J. W. G. Leiper. 1940. Variation in dilution-counts of helminth eggs. J. Helminthol. 18:117-42.

Pipkin, A. C. 1948. The diagnosis of taeniasis by perianal swab. J. Parasitol. 34(Sec. 2):27.

Powell, E. C., and J. B. McCarley. 1975. A murine *Sarcocystis* that causes an *Isospora*-like infection in cats. J. Parasitol. 61:928-31.

Power, I. A. 1971. Helminths of cats from the midwest with a report of *Ancylostoma caninum* in this host. J. Parasitol. 57:610.

Prestwood, A. K. 1971. Cestodes of white-tailed deer *(Odocoileus virginianus)* in the southeastern United States. J. Parasitol. 57:1292.

Pusch, J., I. Senne, and W. Beyer. 1950. An improved, simple method for the identification of parasite eggs in fecal samples. Tieraerztl. Umschau 5:54.

Ratcliffe, H. L. 1944. A method for preparing permanent slides of the ova of parasitic worms. Science 99:394.

Ray, D. K. 1953. Comparative efficiency of zinc sulfate flotation of coccidial cysts of sheep and goats. Proc. Zool. Soc. Bengal. 6:135-38.

Reardon, L. 1938. Studies on oxyuriasis. X. Artifacts in "cellophane" simulating pinworm ova. Am. J. Trop. Med. 18:427-31.

Rees, C. W. 1952. The processing of fecal specimens by the zinc sulfate flotation technique with safeguards for laboratory workers. J. Parasitol. 38(Sec. 2):26.

Regonesi, C., M. Muranda, and J. Artigas. 1954. Técnica del fijador con alcohol polivinílico en el diagnóstico de la amibiasis y otras enteroparasitosis. Bol. Chil. Parasitol. 9:105-9.

Reichenow, E. 1940. Ueber das Kokzid der Equiden, *Globidium leuckarti.* Z. Infektionskr. 56:126-34.

Reid, W. M. 1959. Egg characteristics as aids in species identification and control of chicken tapeworms. Avian Dis. 3:188-97.

———. 1962. Chicken and turkey tapeworms. Handbook to aid in identification and control of tapeworms found in the United States of America. Ga. Agric. Exp. Stn. Bull.

Richardson, V. F., and S. B. Kendall. 1963. Veterinary Protozoology, 3rd ed. F. A. Davis, Philadelphia.

Riley, W. A., and R. O. Christenson. 1931. How to detect the parasites of furbearing animals. Univ. Minn. Agric. Ext. Div. Pamphlet 18.

Ringuelet, R. 1949. Identificación microscópica de los huevos de nematodes comunes en las materias fecales de vacunos, ovinos y equinos. Fasc. C. N. Museo. La Plata, Argentina. Sen. Tec. Did. No. 1:5-25.

Ritchie, L. S., C. Pan, and G. W. Hunter III. 1952. A comparison of the zinc sulfate and the MGL (formalin-ether) technics. J. Parasitol. 38 (Sec. 2):16.

Rivera-Anaya, J. D., and J. Martinez de Jesús. 1952. An improved technique for the microscopic diagnosis of liver fluke infection in cattle. J. Am. Vet. Med. Assoc. 120:203-4.

Roberts, F. H. S., and P. J. O'Sullivan. 1950. Methods for egg counts and larval cultures for strongyles infesting the gastro-intestinal tract of cattle. Aust. J. Agric. Res. 1:99-102.

Roberts, F. H. S., P. J. O'Sullivan, and R. F. Riek. 1951. The significance of faecal egg counts in the diagnosis of parasitic gastro-enteritis of cattle. Aust. Vet. J. 27:17-18.

Roberts, G. A. 1926. Interesting observations in the examination of feces of sucking calves, lambs and pigs (methods and findings). J. Am. Vet. Med. Assoc. 69(n.s. 22):75-79.

Ross, J. G., and J. Armour. 1960. Significance of faecal egg counts and the use of serum albumen levels and packed cell volume percentages to assess pathogenicity of helminthiasis. Vet. Rec. 72:137-39.

Rowan, W. B., and A. L. Gram. 1959. Quantitative recovery of helminth eggs from relatively large samples of feces and sewage. J. Parasitol. 45:615-21.

Rubin, R. 1967. Some observations on the interpretation of fecal egg counts. Am. J. Vet. Clin. Pathol. 1(4):145-48.

Sapero, J. J., and D. K. Lawless. 1953. The MIF stain-preservation technique for the identification of intestinal protozoa. Am. J. Trop. Med. Hyg. 2:613-19.

Sarles, M. P. 1929a. Quantitative studies on the dog and cat hookworm, *Ancylostoma braziliense,* with special emphasis on age resistance. Am. J. Hyg. 10(Sept. suppl.):453-75.

———. 1929b. The effect of age and size of infestation on the egg production of the dog hookworm, *Ancylostoma caninum.* Am. J. Hyg. 10(Nov. suppl.):658-66.

Sawitz, W. 1942. The buoyancy of certain nematode eggs. J. Parasitol. 28:95-102.

Sawitz, W., and E. C. Faust. 1942. The probability of detecting intestinal protozoa by successive stool examinations. Am. J. Trop. Med. 22:131-36.

Sawitz, W., J. E. Tobie, and G. Katz. 1939. The specific gravity of hookworm eggs. Am. J. Trop. Med. 19:171-79.

Schalm, O. W. 1965. Veterinary Hematology, 2nd ed. Lea & Febiger, Philadelphia.

Schnelle, G. B., and T. C. Jones. 1944. Occurrence of the cereal mite in war dogs. J. Am. Vet. Med. Assoc. 104:213-14.

Schuchmann, G., and L. Kieffer. 1922. Ueber den Nachweis von Parasiteneiern im Kote der Haustiere. Berl. Tieraerztl. Wochenschr., Jahrg. 38, Nr. 19, S. 220-21; Nr. 31, S. 357-59.

Scott, J. A. 1937. The effect of various solutions on helminth eggs in feces. J. Parasitol. 23:109-12.

Seddon, H. R., and H. R. Carne. 1927. Incident of coccidiosis in Australian rabbits as determined by faecal examinations. N. S. Wales Dep. Agric. Sci. Bull. 29:33-41.

Seghetti, L. 1950. An improved method of mixing fecal suspensions for nematode egg counts. Proc. Helminthol. Soc. Wash. 17:26-27.

Sheather, A. L. 1923a. Detection of worm eggs in the faeces of animals and some experiences in the treatment of parasitic gastritis in cattle. J. Comp. Pathol. Ther. 36:71-90.

———. 1923b. The detection of intestinal protozoa and mange parasites by a floatation technic. J. Comp. Pathol. Ther. 36:266-75.

———. 1924. The detection of worm eggs and protozoa in the faeces of animals. Vet. Rec. 4:552-57.

Sheffield, H. G., and M. L. Melton. 1970. *Toxoplasma gondii:* The oocyst, sporozoite, and infection of cultured cells. Science 167(3919):892-93.

Shorb, D. A. 1939. Differentiation of eggs of various genera of nematodes parasitic in domestic ruminants in the United States. USDA Tech. Bull. 694.

_____. 1940. A comparative study of the eggs of various species of nematodes parasitic in domestic ruminants. J. Parasitol. 26:223-31.

Shrivastav, J. B. 1954. Comparative efficiency of three different techniques for the diagnosis of cystic forms of intestinal protozoa and helminthic ova in faeces. Indian J. Med. Res. 42:497-508.

Sippel, W. L. 1959. Liver fluke egg counting. Vet. Med. 54:245-46.

Sloss, M. W. 1939. Spurious parasites in a dog. (Sheep parasite ova and oocysts.) Vet. Student (Iowa State Univ.) 1:54.

Smillie, W. G. 1921. A comparison of the number of hookworm ova in the stool with the actual number of hookworms harbored by the individual. Am. J. Trop. Med. 1:389-95.

Sogandares-Bernal, F. 1966. Studies on American paragonimiasis. IV. Observations of the pairing of adult worms in laboratory infections of domestic cats. J. Parasitol. 52:701-3.

Soulsby, E. J. L. 1965. Textbook of Veterinary Clinical Parasitology. F. A. Davis, Philadelphia.

_____. 1968. Helminths, Arthropods and Protozoa of Domesticated Animals (Mönnig), 6th ed. Williams & Wilkins, Baltimore.

Spedding, C. R. W. 1952a. Variations in the egg count of sheep faeces within one day. J. Helminthol. 26:71-86.

_____. 1952b. The value of fecal egg count in sheep. Vet. Rec. 64:813-15.

_____. 1953. Variation in the nematode egg content of sheep feces from day to day. J. Helminthol. 27:9-16.

Spedding, C. R. W., and T. H. Brown. 1956. The "spring rise" in the nematode egg-count of sheep. J. Helminthol. 29:171-78.

Spencer, F. M., and L. S. Monroe. 1961. The Color Atlas of Intestinal Parasites, 1st ed. Charles C Thomas, Springfield, Ill.

Spindler, L. A. 1928. Use of the egg isolation technic in epidemiological studies on ascariasis in Virginia. J. Parasitol. 15:147.

_____. 1929. On the use of a method for the isolation of ascaris eggs from the soil. Am. J. Hyg. 10:157-64.

Steck, W. 1926. A simple direct method for determining the number of worm ova in faeces. Schweiz. Arch. Tierheilkd. 68:561-63.

Steel, E. R. 1930. Routine microscopic fecal examinations in small-animal practice. J. Am. Vet. Med. Assoc. 77 (n.s. 30):9-17.

Stoll, N. R. 1923. Investigations on the control of hookworm disease. XIV. An effective method of counting hookworm eggs in feces. Am. J. Hyg. 3:59-70.

_____. 1930. On methods of counting nematode ova in sheep dung. Parasitology 22:116-36.

Stoll, N. R., and W. C. Hausheer. 1926a. Accuracy in the dilution egg-counting method. Am. J. Hyg. 6(March suppl.):80-133.

_____. 1926b. Concerning two options in dilution egg-counting: Small drop and displacement. Am. J. Hyg. 6(March suppl.):134-45.

Summers, W. A. 1942. A modification of zinc sulphate centrifugal flotation method for recovery of helminth ova in formalinized feces. J. Parasitol. 28:345-46.

Swanson, L. E., and H. H. Hopper. 1950. Diagnosis of liver fluke infection in cattle. J. Am. Vet. Med. Assoc. 117:127-29.

Swartzwelder, J. C. 1939. A comparison of five laboratory techniques for the demonstration of intestinal parasites. J. Trop. Med. Hyg. 42:185-87.

Taylor, E. L. 1934. A method of estimating the number of worms present in the fourth stomach and small intestine of sheep and cattle for the definite diagnosis of parasitic gastritis. Vet. Rec. 14:474-76.

_____. 1935. Seasonal fluctuation in the number of eggs of trichostrongylid worms in the faeces of ewes. J. Parasitol. 21:175-79.

_____. 1939. Diagnosis of helminthiasis by means of egg counts, with special reference to red-worm disease in horses. Vet. Rec. 51:895-98.

Telemann, W. 1908. Eine Methode zur Erleichterung der Auffindung von Parasiteneiern in den Faeces. Dtsch. Med. Wochenschr. 34:1510-11.

Tetley, J. H. 1941a. Haemonchus contortus eggs: Comparison of those in utero with those recovered from feces, and a statistical method for identifying H. contortus eggs in mixed infections. J. Parasitol. 27:453-63.

_____. 1941b. The differentiation of eggs of the trichostrongylid species Nematodirus filicollis and N. spathiger. J. Parasitol. 27:473-80.

_____. 1949. Rhythms in nematode parasitism of sheep. N.Z. Dep. Sci. Ind. Res. Bull. 96.

Teuscher, E. 1957. Eine neue praktische Flotationsmethode für den koprologischen Nachweis der Leberegeleier. Schweiz. Arch. Tierheilkd. 99:523-28.

Teuscher, E., and G. Schuler. 1959. Weitere Untersuchungen zur koprologischen diagnose der Fasciolose bei Wiederkäuren. Schweiz. Arch. Tierheilkd. 101:331-36.

Tobie, J. E., L. V. Reardon, J. Bozicevich, Bao-Chih Shih, N. Mantel, and E. H. Thomas. 1951. The efficiency of the zinc sulfate technic in the detection of intestinal protozoa by successive stool examinations. Ann. Trop. Med. 31:552-60.

Todd, K. S., Jr., N. D. Levine, and P. A. Boatman. 1976. Effect of desiccation on the survival of infective *Haemonchus contortus* larvae under laboratory conditions. J. Parasitol. 62:247-49.

Turner, J. H. 1951. Counting *Nematodirus spathiger* eggs in sheep dung. Proc. Helminthol. Soc. Wash. 18:132-35.

Turner, J. H., and G. I. Wilson. 1961. Experimental strongyloidiasis in sheep and goats. V. Effect of certain environmental conditions and chemicals on the infective larvae of *Strongyloides papillosus*. J. Parasitol. 47:30.

Ubelaker, J. E., and V. F. Allison. 1975. Scanning electron microscopy of the eggs of *Ascaris lumbricoides*, *A. suum*, *Toxocara canis*, and *T. mystax*. J. Parasitol. 61:802-7.

Vajda, T. 1922. A new method for detecting the eggs of parasites in feces. J. Am. Vet. Med. Assoc. 61 (n.s. 14):534-36.

Vanparijs, O. F. J., and D. C. Thienpont. 1973. Canine and feline helminth and protozoan infections in Belgium. J. Parasitol. 59:327-30.

Vogelsang, E. G. 1957. Diagnostico microscopico de la distomatosis bovina. Rev. Med. Vet. Parasitol. (Maracay) 16:33-38.

Watson, J. M. 1947. A modification of the zinc sulfate centrifugal flotation technique for the concentration of helminth ova and protozoan cysts in faeces. Ann. Trop. Med. Parasitol. 41:43-45.

Webster, G. 1958. On prenatal infection and the migration of *Toxocara canis*, Werner 1782, in dogs. Can. J. Zool. 36:435-40.

White, E. G. 1955. The eggs of *Hyostrongylus rubidus*, Hall 1921, a stomach worm of the pig, and their recognition in pig faeces. Br. Vet. J. 111:11-15.

Whitlock, H. V. 1941. A new apparatus for counting small numbers of nematode eggs in faeces. Aust. Counc. Sci. Ind. Res. J. 14:306-7.

————. 1942. The preparation and examination of faecal cultures for the differentiation of larvae of sheep nematodes. Aust. Counc. Sci. Ind. Res. J. 15:56-58.

————. 1943. A method of preventing the development of strongylid eggs in sheep faeces during transport and storage. Aust. Counc. Sci. Ind. Res. J. 16:215-16.

————. 1948. Some modifications of the McMaster helminth egg-counting technique and apparatus. Aust. Counc. Sci. Ind. Res. J. 21:177-80.

————. 1950. A technique for counting trematode eggs in sheep faeces. J. Helminthol. 24:47-52.

————. 1959. The recovery and identification of the first stage larvae of sheep nematodes. Aust. Vet. J. 35:310-16.

Whitlock, J. H. 1941. A practical dilution-egg-count procedure. J. Am. Vet. Med. Assoc. 98:466-69.

Whitney, L. F. 1936. A study of 1,000 fecal examination reports. Vet. Med. 31:104.

Widgor, M. 1919. A study of the fecal examinations of 1,000 imported dogs. J. Am. Vet. Med. Assoc. 56(n.s. 9):189-91.

Willis, H. H. 1921. A simple levitation method for the detection of hookworm ova. Med. J. Aust. 8:375-76; 7th Ann. Rep., Rockefeller Found. Int. Health Board, 1920.

Willmott, S., and F. R. N. Pester. 1952. Variations in faecal egg-counts in paramphistome infections as determined by a new technique. J. Helminthol. 26:147-56.

Wilson, G. I. 1957. Comparison of the DCF and McMaster egg-counting techniques as applied to nematode parasitism of sheep. J. Parasitol. 43(Sec. 2):20.

Wilson, I. D. 1934. Sodium chloride vs. cane sugar for parasite egg flotation. Cornell Vet. 24:79-80.

Winn, M. M., A. P. Moon, S. S. Lin, S. Asakura, and H. Yoshida. 1957. The effect of changes in pH and specific gravity on the recovery of certain helminth eggs and protozoan cysts in the formalin-ether (406th MGL) fecal concentration technique. J. Parasitol. 43(Sec. 2):41.

Worley, D. E., and R. H. Jacobson. 1970. *Physaloptera* sp. in domestic sheep in Montana. J. Parasitol. 56:840.

Wright, P. D., and F. L. Anderson. 1972. Parasitic helminths of sheep and cattle in central Utah. J. Parasitol. 58:959.

Wycoff, D. E., and L. S. Ritchie. 1952. Efficiency of the formalin-ether concentration technic. J. Parasitol. 38(Sec. 2):15–16.

Wycoff, D. E., L. P. Frick, and L. S. Ritchie. 1958. Statistical evaluation of the formalin-ether (406th MGL) fecal sedimentation concentration procedure. Am. J. Trop. Med. Hyg. 7:150–57.

Zawadowsky, M. M., and S. N. Zvjaguintzev. 1933. The seasonal fluctuations in the number of eggs of *Nematodirus* sp. in feces. J. Parasitol. 19:269–79.

REFERENCES FOR SECTION 2

Anderson, R. C. 1956. Life cycle and seasonal transmission of *Ornithofilaria fallisensis* Anderson, a parasite of domestic and wild ducks. Can. J. Zool. 34:485–525.

Atchley, F. O. 1951. *Leucocytozoon andrewsi* n. sp., from chickens observed in a survey of blood parasites in domestic animals in South Carolina. J. Parasitol. 37:483–88.

Becker, E. R., W. F. Hollander, and W. H. Pattillo. 1956. Naturally occurring *Plasmodium* and *Haemoproteus* infection in the common pigeon. J. Parasitol. 42:474–78.

Becker, E. R., W. F. Hollander, and J. H. Farmer. 1957. Occurrence (1956) of *Haemoproteus sacharovi* and *Plasmodium relictum* in a central Iowa pigeon colony. Proc. Iowa Acad. Sci. 64:648–49.

Belding, D. L. 1958. Basic Clinical Parasitology. Appleton-Century-Crofts, New York.

Bell, F. N. 1934. A microfilaria in the blood of cattle. J. Am. Vet. Med. Assoc. 85(n.s. 38):747–59. *(Setaria cervi)*

Benjamin, M. M. 1961. Outline of Veterinary Clinical Pathology. Iowa State Univ. Press, Ames.

Benjamin, M. M., and W. V. Lumb. 1959. *Haemobartonella canis* infection in a dog. J. Am. Vet. Med. Assoc. 135:388–90.

Bennett, G. F. 1962. The hematocrit centrifuge for laboratory diagnosis of hematozoa. Can. J. Zool. 40:124–25.

Berrier, H. H. 1958. Diagnostic Aids in the Practice of Veterinary Medicine. C. W. Alban, St. Louis.

Bierer, B. W. 1950. Leucocytozoon infection in turkeys. Vet. Med. 45:87–88.

Briggs, N. T. 1960. Comparison of *Leucocytozoon simondi* in Pekin and Muscovy ducklings. Proc. Helminthol. Soc. Wash. 27:151–56.

Burch, G. R., and H. E. Blair. 1951. A rapid test for the diagnosis of *Dirofilaria immitis*. Vet. Med. 46:128–30.

Cameron, T. W. M. 1952. The Parasites of Domestic Animals. J. B. Lippincott, Philadelphia.

Carlos, E. R., and A. C. Directo. 1960. Clinical trial of dichlorophenarsine hydrochloride in treatment of canine heartworm infection. J. Am. Vet. Med. Assoc. 137:717–20. (Ohishi's diagnostic technique)

Carr, D. T., and H. E. Essex. 1944. Bartonellosis: A cause of severe anemia in splenectomized dogs. Proc. Soc. Exp. Biol. Med. 57:44–5.

Chernin, E., and E. H. Sadun. 1949. *Leucocytozoon simondi* infections in domestic ducks in northern Michigan, with a note on *Haemoproteus*. Poult. Sci. 28:890–93.

Christensen, B. M., and W. N. Andrews. 1976. Natural infection of *Aedes trivittatus* (Coq.) with *Dirofilaria immitis* in central Iowa. J. Parasitol. 62:276–80.

Chularerk, P., and R. S. Desowitz. 1970. A simplified membrane filtration technique for the diagnosis of microfilaremia. J. Parasitol. 56:623–24.

Coatney, G. R. 1938. A strain of *Plasmodium relictum* from doves and pigeons infective to canaries and the common fowl. Am. J. Hyg. 27:380.

Coatney, G. R., and E. West. 1940. Studies on *Haemoproteus sacharovi* of mourning doves and pigeons, with notes on *H. maccallumi*. Am. J. Hyg. 31(Sec. C):9–13.

Coffin, D. L. 1953. Manual of Veterinary Clinical Pathology, 3rd ed. Comstock, Ithaca, N.Y.

Collins, R. C. 1973. Onchocerciasis of horses in southeastern Louisiana. J. Parasitol. 59:1016–20.

Collins, W. E., G. M. Jeffrey, J. C. Skinner, A. J. Harrison, and F. Arnold. 1966. Blood parasites of birds at Wateree, South Carolina. J. Parasitol. 52:671–73.

Cook, A. R. 1954. Gametocyte development of *Leucytozoon simondi*. Proc. Helminthol. Soc. Wash. 21:1–9.

Crawley, H. 1912. *Trypanosoma americanum*, a common blood parasite of American cattle. USDA Bur. Anim. Ind. Bull. 145. *(Trypanosoma theileri)*

Crocker, K. W., and M. D. Sutter. 1954. Bovine eperythrozoonosis. Vet. Med. 49:305–6.

De Kock, G., and J. Quinlan. 1926. Difference between *Anaplasma* and Jolly bodies. S. Afr. J. Sci. 23:755–59.

Dennis, D. T., and B. H. Kean. 1971. Isolation of microfilariae: Report of a new method. J. Parasitol. 57:1146.

Dicke, W. E. 1934. Anaplasmosis-like disease in swine. Vet. Med. 29:288. (Eperythrozoonosis)

Donahoe, J. M. R. 1975. Experimental infection of cats with *Dirofilaria immitis*. J. Parasitol. 61:599–605.

Donovan, E. F., and W. F. Loeb. 1960. Haemobartonellosis in the dog. Vet. Med. 55:57–62.

Doyle, L. P. 1932. A rickettsia-like or anaplasmosis-like disease in swine. J. Am. Vet. Med. Assoc. 81(n.s. 34):668–71.

Drake, C. J., and R. M. Jones. 1930. The pigeon fly and pigeon malaria in Iowa. Iowa State J. Sci. 4:253–61. (Haemoproteosis)

Eberhard, M. L., and W. G. Winkler. 1974. *Onchocerciasis* among ungulate animals in Georgia. J. Parasitol. 60:971.

Eichenwald, H. F. 1957. The laboratory diagnosis of toxoplasmosis. Ann. N.Y. Acad. Sci. 64(Art. 2):207–14.

Field, J. W. 1941. Further note on a method of staining malarial parasites in thick blood films. R. Soc. Trop. Med. Hyg. 35:35–42. (Field's stain)

Flint, J. C., and D. H. McKelvie. 1956. Feline infectious anemia: Diagnosis and treatment. 1955. Proc. Am. Vet. Med. Assoc., pp. 240–42. (*Haemobartonella felis* n. sp.)

Flint, J. C., M. H. Roepke, and R. Jensen. 1958. Feline infectious anemia. I. Clinical aspects. Am. J. Vet. Res. 19:164–68. (Haemobartonellosis)

Foil, L., and T. C. Orihel. 1975. *Dirofilaria immitis* (Leidy, 1856) in the beaver, *Castor canadensis*. J. Parasitol. 61:433.

Foote, L. E., W. E. Brock, and B. Gallaher. 1951. Ictero-anemia, eperythrozoonosis, an anaplasmosis-like disease of swine proved to be caused by a filtrable virus. North Am. Vet. 32:17–23.

Fukamachi, H. 1960. Experimental studies on the periodicity of microfilariae. Endem. Dis. Bull. Nagasaki Univ. 2:27–38.

Gates, D. W., and T. O. Roby. 1956. Status of the complement-fixation test for the diagnosis of anaplasmosis in 1955. Ann. N.Y. Acad. Sci. 64(Art. 2):31–39.

Glaser, R. W. 1922. A study of *Trypanosoma americanum*. J. Parasitol. 8:136–44. (*Trypanosoma theileri*)

Graham, J. M. 1974. Canine filariasis in northeastern Kansas. J. Parasitol. 60:322–26.

——. 1975. Filariasis in coyotes from Kansas and Colorado. J. Parasitol. 61:513–16.

Griesemer, R. A. 1958. Bartonellosis. J. U.S. Natl. Cancer Inst. 20:949–54. (Haemobartonellosis)

Hepler, O. E. 1960. Manual of Clinical Laboratory Methods, 4th ed. Charles C Thomas, Springfield, Ill.

Herman, C. M. 1954. *Haemoproteus* infection in waterfowl. Proc. Helminthol. Soc. Wash. 21:37–42.

Hewitt, R. 1940. Bird malaria. Am. J. Hyg., Monogr. Ser. 15. (*Plasmodium* spp.)

Hinman, E. H. 1935. Studies on the dog heartworm, *Dirofilaria immitis* with special reference to filarial periodicity. Am. J. Trop. Med. 15:371–84.

Hoare, C. A. 1923. An experimental study of the sheep-trypanosome (*T. melophagium* Flu, 1908), and its transmission by the sheep-ked (*Melophagus ovinus* L.). Parasitology 15:365–424.

Hofstad, M. S., B. W. Calnek, C. F. Helmboldt, W. Malcolm Reid, H. W. Yoder (eds). 1978. Diseases of Poultry, 7th ed. Iowa State University Press, Ames.

Jacobs, L. 1956. Propagation, morphology and biology of *Toxoplasma*. Ann. N.Y. Acad. Sci. 64(Art. 2):154–79.

Johnson, E. P. 1942. Further observations on a blood protozoon of turkeys transmitted by *Simulium nigroparvum* (Twinn). Am. J. Vet. Res. 3:214–18. (*Leucocytozoon smithi*)

Kikuth, W. 1928. Ueber einen neuen Anämieerreger, Bartonella canis, nov. sp. Klin. Wochenschr. 7:1729–30. (*Haemobartonella canis*)

Kingston, N., and J. Morton. 1973. Trypanosomes from elk (*Cervys canadensis*) in Wyoming. J. Parasitol. 59:1132–33.

Knott, J. I. 1939. Method for making microfilarial surveys on day blood. Trans. R. Soc. Trop. Med. Hyg. 33:191–96.

Koutz, F. R. 1957. *Demodex folliculorum* studies. VI. The internal phase of canine demodectic mange. J. Am. Vet. Med. Assoc. 131:45–48.

Krinsky, W. L., and L. L. Pechuman. 1975. Trypanosomes in horse flies and deer flies in central New York State. J. Parasitol. 61:12–16.

Lapage, G. 1956. Veterinary Parasitology. Charles C Thomas, Springfield, Ill.

Levine, N. D. 1973. Protozoan Parasites of Domestic Animals and of Man, 2nd ed. Burgess, Minneapolis.

Levine, N. D., and S. Kantor. 1959. Checklist of blood parasites of the order Columbiformes. Wildl. Dis. 1:1–38. (Microfiche)

Levine, N. D., A. M. Watrach, S. Kantor, and H. J. Hardenbrook. 1956. A case of bovine trypanosomiasis due to *Trypanosoma theileri* in Illinois. J. Parasitol. 42:553.

Live, I., and E. L. Stubbs. 1938. Diagnosis of filariasis in the dog. J. Am. Vet. Med. Assoc. 92(n.s. 45):686–89.

Lotze, J. C., and G. W. Bowman. 1942. Occurrence of *Bartonella* in cases of anaplasmosis and in apparently normal cattle. Proc. Helminthol. Soc. Wash. 9:71–72. *(Haemobartonella bovis)*

Lotze, J. C., and M. J. Yiengst. 1941. "Eperythrozoonosis" in cattle in the United States. North Am. Vet. 22:345–46.

_____. 1942. Studies on the nature of *Anaplasma*. Am. J. Vet. Res. 3:312–20.

Lucas, A. M., and C. Jamroz. 1961. Atlas of Avian Hematology. USDA Monogr. 25.

Manwell, R. D. 1938. The identification of the avian malarias. Am. J. Trop. Med. 18:565–75.

Marquardt, W. C., and W. E. Fabian. 1966. The distribution in Illinois of filariids of dogs. J. Parasitol. 52:318–22.

Mathey, W. R. 1955. Two cases of *Plasmodium relictum* infection in domestic pigeons in the Sacramento area. Vet. Med. 50:318.

Melvin, D. M., and M. M. Brooke. 1955. Triton X-100 in Giemsa staining of blood parasites. Stain Tech. 30:269–75.

Meyer, M. C., and L. R. Penner. 1958. Laboratory Essentials of Animal Parasitology. W. C. Brown, Dubuque, Iowa.

Morehouse, N. F. 1945. The occurrence of *Haemoproteus* sp. in the domesticated turkey. Trans. Am. Microsc. Soc. 64:109–11.

Morgan, B. B., and P. A. Hawkins. 1952. Veterinary Protozoology, 2nd ed. Burgess, Minneapolis.

Morris, M. L., J. H. Dinkel, and D. F. Green. 1935a. Laboratory diagnosis of dog heartworms. North Am. Vet. 16(9):34.

_____. 1935b. Comparative study of the drop method and concentration method for the diagnosis of *Dirofilaria immitis*. North Am. Vet. 16(11):39–40.

Muller, G. H., and R. W. Kirk. 1969. Small Animal Dermatology. W. B. Saunders, Philadelphia.

Neveu-Lemaire, M. 1943. Traité de Protozoologie Médicale et Vétérinaire. Vigot Frères, Paris.

Newberne, J. W. 1955. Pathology of *Leucocytozoon* infection in turkeys with a note on its tissue stages. Am. J. Vet. Res. 16:593–97.

_____. 1957. Studies on the histopathology of *Leucocytozoon simondi* infection. Am. J. Vet. Res. 18:191–99.

Newton, W. L., and W. H. Wright. 1956. Occurrence of a dog filariid other than *Dirofilaria immitis* in the United States. J. Parasitol. 42:246–58. (*Dipetalonema* sp.)

_____. 1957. Reevaluation of the canine filariasis problem in the United States. Vet. Med. 52:75–78.

New York Academy of Sciences. 1956. Some protozoan diseases of man and animals: Anaplasmosis, babesiosis, and toxoplasmosis. N.Y. Acad. Sci. Ann. 64(Art. 2):25–277.

Norman, L., and A. W. Donaldson. 1955. Spores of helicosporous fungi resembling microfilariae in blood films. Am. J. Trop. Med. Hyg. 4:889–93.

O'Roke, E. C. 1934. A malaria-like disease of ducks caused by *Leucocytozoon anatis*. Univ. Mich. Sch. Forest. Conserv. Bull. 4.

Otto, G. F., and P. M. Bauman. 1959. Canine filariasis. Vet. Med. 54:87–96. (*Dirofilaria* and *Dipetalonema*)

Pacheco, G. 1966. Progressive changes in certain serological responses to *Dirofilaria immitis* infection in the dog. J. Parasitol. 52:311–17.

Rees, C. W. 1930. Fixing thin blood smears for staining with iron hematoxylin and with Giemsa's stain, especially for Texas fever. Science 71:134. *(Babesia bigemina)*

_____. 1934. Characteristics of the piroplasms *Babesia argentina* and *B. bigemina* in the United States. J. Agric. Res. 48:427–38.

Rhoads, C. P., and D. K. Miller. 1935. The association of *Bartonella* bodies with induced anemia in the dog. J. Exp. Med. 61:139–48.

Richardson, U. F., and S. B. Kendall. 1958. Veterinary Protozoology, 2nd ed. Oliver and Boyd, London.

Ristic, M. 1960. Studies of anaplasmosis. Filtration of the causative agent. Am. J. Vet. Res. 21:890-94.

———. 1962. A capillary tube-agglutination test for anaplasmosis — A preliminary report. J. Am. Vet. Med. Assoc. 141:588-94.

Ristic, M., F. H. White, and D. A. Sanders. 1957. Detection of *Anaplasma marginale* by means of fluorescein-labeled antibody. Am. J. Vet. Res. 18:924-31.

Rothstein, N. 1958. Vital staining of blood parasites with acridine orange. J. Parasitol. 44:588-94.

Rothstein, N., and M. L. Brown. 1960. Vital staining and differentiation of microfilariae. Am. J. Vet. Res. 21:1090-94.

Runnells, R. A., W. S. Monlux, and A. W. Monlux. 1965. Principles of Veterinary Pathology, 7th ed. Iowa State Univ. Press, Ames.

Saunders, D. A. 1937. Observations on canine babesiasis (piroplasmosis). J. Am. Vet. Med. Assoc. 90(n.s. 43):27-40.

Savage, A., and J. M. Isa. 1945. An outbreak of *Leucocytozoon* disease in turkeys. Cornell Vet. 35:270-72.

———. 1958. A picture of *Eperythrozoon suis*. Cornell Vet. 48:10-11.

———. 1959. A note on *Leucocytozoon* disease in ducks. Cornell Vet. 49:252-54.

Scarborough, R. A. 1930-32. The blood picture of normal laboratory animals. Yale J. Biol. Med. 3:63-80, 169-79, 267-82, 359-73, 431-40, 547-52; 4:69-82, 199-206, 323-44.

Schalm, O. W. 1965. Veterinary Hematology. Lea & Febiger, Philadelphia.

Schillhorn van Veen, Tj. W., and C. Blotkamp. 1972. A rapid staining method for microfilariae. J. Parasitol. 58:446.

Schnelle, G. B., and R. M. Young. 1944. Clinical studies on microfilarial periodicity in war dogs. Bull. U.S. Army Med. Dep. 80:52.

Schwartzman, R. M., and E. D. Besch. 1958. Feline infectious anemia. Vet. Med. 53:494-500. *(Haemobartonella felis)*

Seibold, H. R., and W. S. Bailey. 1957. Babesiasis (piroplasmosis) in dogs. J. Am. Vet. Med. Assoc. 130:46-48.

Simpson, C. F., and J. H. Green. 1959. Cultivation of *Trypanosoma theileri* in liquid medium at 37 C. Cornell Vet. 49:192-93.

Smith, H. A., and T. C. Jones. 1957. Veterinary Pathology. Lea & Febiger, Philadelphia.

Splitter, E. J. 1950a. *Theileria mutans* associated with bovine anaplasmosis in the United States. J. Am. Vet. Med. Assoc. 117:134-35. *(Gonderia mutans)*

———. 1950b. *Eperythrozoon suis* n. sp. and *E. parvum* n. sp., two new blood parasites of swine. Science 111:513-14.

———. 1950c. *Eperythrozoon suis*, the etiologic agent of ictero-anemia or an anaplasmosis-like disease in swine. Am. J. Vet. Res. 11:324-30.

———. 1958. Complement-fixation test in the diagnosis of eperythrozoonosis in swine. J. Am. Vet. Med. Assoc. 132:47-49.

Splitter, E. J., and R. L. Williamson. 1950. Eperythrozoonosis in swine: A preliminary report. J. Am. Vet. Med. Assoc. 116:360-64.

Splitter, E. J., H. D. Anthony, and M. J. Twiehaus. 1956a. *Anaplasma ovis* in the United States. Am. J. Vet. Res. 17:487-91.

Splitter, E. J., E. D. Castro, and W. L. Kanawyer. 1956b. Feline infectious anemia. Vet. Med. 51:17-22. (Haemobartonellosis)

Stubbs, E. L., and I. Live. 1935. Diagnosis of filariasis in the dog. J. Am. Vet. Med. Assoc. 87(n.s. 40):680-82.

Thrasher, J. P., K. G. Gould, M. J. Lynch, and C. C. Harris. 1968. Filarial infections of dogs in Atlanta, Georgia. J. Am. Vet. Med. Assoc. 153(8):1059-63.

Travis, B. V. 1939. Preliminary note on the occurrence of *Leucocytozoon smithi* Laveran and Lucet (1905) in turkeys in the southwestern United States. J. Parasitol. 25:278.

Turner, A. W., and D. Murnane. 1930. On the presence of the non-pathogenic *Trypanosoma melophagium* in the blood of Victorian sheep, and its transmission by *Melophagus ovinus*. Aust. J. Exp. Biol. Med. Sci. 7:5-8.

Underwood, P. C., and P. D. Harwood. 1939. Survival and location of the microfilariae of *Dirofilaria immitis* in the dog. J. Parasitol. 25:23-33.

United States Department of Agriculture, and State Agricultural Experiment Stations. 1957. Proc. 3rd Natl. Res. Conf. Anaplasmosis in Cattle. Kansas State Univ., Manhattan.

Votava, C. L., and P. E. Thompson. 1973. *Onchocerca lienalis* of cattle in Georgia. J. Parasitol. 59:938-39.

Wallenstein, W. L., and B. J. Tibola. 1960. Survey of canine filariasis in a Maryland area. Incidence of *Dirofilaria immitis* and *Dipetalonema*. J. Am. Vet. Med. Assoc. 137:712-16.

Walton, B. C., and I. Arjona. 1971. Utilization of whole blood specimens on filter paper for the indirect fluorescent antibody test for toxoplasmosis. J. Parasitol. 57:678–80.

Weinman, D. 1944. Infectious anemias due to *Bartonella* and related red blood cell parasites. Trans. Am. Philosoph. Soc. 33:243–51. (Haemobartonellosis)

West, J. L., and L. E. Starr. 1940. Further observations on a blood protozoan infection in turkeys. Vet. Med. 35:649–53. *(Leucocytozoon smithi)*

Whitlock, J. H. 1960. Diagnosis of Veterinary Parasitisms. Lea & Febiger, Philadelphia. (no protozoa)

Williams, J. R., and A. W. Dade. 1976. *Dirofilaria immitis* infection in a wolverine. J. Parasitol. 62:174–75.

Winter, H. 1959. Pathology of canine dirofilariasis. Am. J. Vet. Res. 20:366–71.

Wongsathuaythong, S. 1961. Detection of microfilariae in peripheral blood of monkeys by the microcapillary technique. J. Trop. Med. Hyg. 64:255–57.

Yaeger, R. C. 1960. A method for isolating trypanosomes from blood. J. Parasitol. 46:288.

REFERENCES FOR SECTION 3

Armitage, F. D. 1936. A method for the preparation of mange mites for microscopical examination. Vet. Rec. 48:1404–6.

Baker, D. W. 1946. Barn itch. Parasitol. Lab., Vet. Exp. Stn., Cornell Univ.

Baker, E. W., and G. W. Wharton. 1952. An Introduction to Acarology. Macmillan, New York.

Baker, E. W., T. M. Evans, D. J. Gould, W. B. Hull, and H. L. Keegan. 1956. A Manual of Parasitic Mites of Medical or Economic Importance. Natl. Pest Control Assoc., New York.

Baker, E. W., J. H. Camin, F. Cunliff, T. A. Wooley, and C. E. Yunker. 1958. Guide to the Families of Mites. Inst. Acarology, Univ. of Md., College Park.

Barker, R. W., A. L. Hoch, R. G. Buckner, and J. A. Hair. 1973. Hematological changes in white-tailed deer fawns, *Odocoileus virginianus*, infested with Theileria-infected lone star ticks. J. Parasitol. 59:1091–98.

Bell, D. S., W. D. Pounder, B. H. Edgington, and O. G. Bentley. 1952. *Psorergates ovis*, a cause of itchiness in sheep. J. Am. Vet. Med. Assoc. 120:117–20.

Benbrook, E. A. 1929. Skin examination of domestic animals for evidence of parasitic mites. Iowa State Coll. Vet. Pract. Bull. 9, pp. 37–56.

Besch, E. D. 1960. Notes on the morphology of *Pneumonyssoides caninum* (Chandler and Ruhe, 1940) Fain, 1955 (Acarina: Halarachnidae). J. Parasitol. 46:351–54.

Bingham, M. L. 1944. Some clinical diagnostic methods of use in conditions associated with animal parasites. Vet. Rec. 56:313–16.

Brennan, J., and J. T. Reed. 1973. More new genera and species of chiggers (Acarina: Trombiculidae) from Venezuela. J. Parasitol. 59:706–10.

Burrichter, D. 1966. Sarcoptic mange in a calf. Iowa State Univ. Vet. 28(3):121–23.

Carter, H. B. 1941. A skin disease of sheep due to an ectoparasitic mite, *Psorergates ovis* Womersley. Aust. Vet. J. 17:193–201.

Chandler, W. L., and D. S. Ruhe. 1940. *Pneumonyssus caninum* n. sp., a mite from the frontal sinus of the dog. J. Parasitol. 26:59–67.

Chapin, E. A. 1925. *Freyana (Microspalax) chaneyi* from a turkey, *Meleagris gallopavo.* J. Parasitol. 12:113.

Clark, J. D., and Hyong-Sun Ah. 1976. *Cheyletiella parasitivorax* (Megnin) a parasitic mite causing mange in the domestic rabbit. J. Parasitol. 62:125.

Cooper, K. W. 1946. The occurrence of the mite *Cheyletiella parasitivorax* (Mégnin) in North America, with notes on its synonymy and "parasitic" habit. J. Parasitol. 32:480–82.

Cram, E. B. 1925. Demodectic mange of the goat in the United States. J. Am. Vet. Med. Assoc. 66(n.s. 19):475–80.

Crawley, H. 1922. A case of demodectic mange in a bull. J. Am. Vet. Med. Assoc. 61(n.s. 14):441–43.

Crossley, D. A., Jr. 1950. A new species of nasal mite, *Neonyssus columbae* from the pigeon. Proc. Entomol. Soc. Wash. 52:309–12.

———. 1952. Two new nasal mites from columbiform birds. J. Parasitol. 38:385–90. *(Speleognathus striatus)*

Dakin, G. W. 1956. An outbreak of *Trombicula autumnalis* infestation in dogs. Vet Rec. 68:331. (Chigger mite)

Davis, J. W. 1954. Studies of the sheep mite, *Psorergates ovis*. Am. J. Vet. Res. 15:255–57.

Desh, C., and W. B. Nutting. 1972. *Demodex folliculorum* (Simon) *D. brevis akbulatova* of man: Redescription and reevaluation. J. Parasitol. 58:169–77.
Douglas, J. R. 1951. New parasite records from California dogs. Cornell Vet. 41:342–46. *(Pneumonyssus caninum)*
Ewing, H. E. 1944. The Trombiculid mites (chigger mites) and their relation to disease. J. Parasitol. 30:339–65.
Ewing, H. E., and A. Hartzell. 1918. The chigger mites affecting man and domestic animals. J. Econ. Entomol. 11:256–64.
Fisher, W. F. 1973. Natural transmission of *Demodex bovis* Stiles in cattle. J. Parasitol. 59:223.
Friedman, R. 1942. Biology of *Acarus scabiei*. Froben Press, New York.
Frost, R. C., and W. P. Beresford-Jones. 1958. Otodectic mange in the dog. Vet. Rec. 70:740–42.
Furman, D. P. 1954. A revision of the genus *Pneumonyssus* (Acarina: Halarachnidae). J. Parasitol. 40:31–42.
Gaafar, S. M., H. E. Smalley, and R. D. Turk. 1958. Incidence of Demodex species on skins of apparently normal dogs. J. Am. Vet. Med. Assoc. 133:122–23.
Greve, J. H., and S. M. Gaafar. 1966. Natural transmission of *Demodex canis* in dogs. J. Am. Vet. Med. Assoc. 148:1043–45.
Greve, J. H., V. S. Myers, and M. W. Sloss. 1964. Chorioptic dermatitis in a horse. Iowa State Univ. Vet. 27:68–70.
Hardenbergh, J. G., and C. H. Schlotthauer. 1925. Demodectic mange of the goat and its treatment. J. Am. Vet. Med. Assoc. 67(n.s. 20):486–89.
Hering, E. A. 1845. Eine neue Kratzmilbe *(Sarcoptes bovis)*. Jahresh. Ver. Vaterl. Naturk. Wurttemberg 1:110–14.
Himonas, C. A., J. Theodorides, and A. E. Alexakes. 1975. Demodectic mites in the eyelids of domestic animals in Greece. J. Parasitol. 61:767.
Hirst, S. 1922. Mites injurious to domestic animals. Br. Mus. Econ. Ser. 13:1–107.
———. 1924. On a new mite of the genus *Chorioptes* parasitic on goats in the United States. Ann. Mag. Nat. Hist. 13:538. *(Chorioptes texanus)*
Hollander, W. F. 1956. Acarids of domestic pigeons. Trans. Am. Microsc. Soc. 75:461–80.
Hoyer's solution for mounting mites. *In:* Baker, E. W., and G. W. Wharton. 1952. Introduction to Acarology. Macmillan, New York, p. 10.
Hull, W. B. 1956. Nymphal stages of *Pneumonyssus simicola* Banks, 1901 (Acarina: Halarachnidae). J. Parasitol. 42:653–56.
Hwang, J. C. 1959. Case report of the quill mite, *Syringophilus bipectinatus* in poultry. Proc. Helminthol. Soc. Wash. 26:47–50.
James, W. A., R. Graham, and F. Thorp. 1930. Epidermoptic scabies in a hen. J. Am. Vet. Med. Assoc. 76:93.
Koutz, F. R. 1953. *Demodex folliculorum* studies. II. Comparison of various diagnostic methods. Speculum 6:8–9, 23, 26, 55.
———. 1955a. Life cycle, diagnosis, and treatment of various mites that attack small animals. Vet. Med. 50:278–81.
———. 1955b. *Demodex folliculorum* studies. V. Demodectic mange in cattle. Vet. Med. 50:305–6; 330.
———. 1957. *Demodex folliculorum* studies. VI. The internal phase of canine demodectic mange. J. Am. Vet. Med. Assoc. 131:45–48.
Koutz, F. R., D. M. Chamberlain, and C. R. Cole. 1953. *Pneumonyssus caninum* in the nasal cavity and paranasal sinuses. J. Am. Vet. Med. Assoc. 122:106–9.
Koutz, F. R., H. F. Groves, and C. M. Gee. 1960. Survey of *Demodex canis* in the skin of clinically normal dogs. Vet. Med. 55(8):52–53.
Lapage, G. 1956. Veterinary Parasitology. Charles C Thomas, Springfield, Ill.
Lapage, G., ed. 1956. Mönnig's Veterinary Helminthology and Entomology, 4th ed. Williams & Wilkins, Baltimore.
———. 1962. Mönnig's Veterinary Helminthology and Entomology, 5th ed. Williams & Wilkins, Baltimore.
Lavoipierre, M. M. J. 1953. The undescribed male and female of the pigeon mite, *Syringophilus columbae* Hirst, 1920. Trans. R. Soc. Trop. Med. Hyg. 47:7.
Lebel, R. R., and W. B. Nutting. 1973. Demodectic mites of subhuman primates. I. *Demodex saimiri* sp. n. (Acari: Demodicidae) from the squirrel monkey, *Saimiri sciureus*. J. Parasitol. 59:719–22.
Leidy, J. 1872. On a mite in the ear of the ox. Proc. Acad. Nat. Sci. Phila., p. 9.
Little, R. B. 1932. Demodectic (follicular) mange in cattle. J. Am. Vet. Med. Assoc. 80(n.s. 33):922–26.

Martin, H. M., and M. J. Deubler. 1943. Acariasis of the upper respiratory tract of the dog. Univ. Pa. Vet. Ext. Quart. 89:21-27.

Meleney, W. P., and I. H. Roberts. 1970. *Otobius megnini* (Acarina: Argasidae) in the ears of pronghorn antelope *(Antilocapra americana)* in New Mexico. J. Parasitol. 917.

Menzies, G. C. 1957. The cattle ear mite, *Raillietia auris* (Leidy, 1872) in Texas. J. Parasitol. 43:200.

Monlux, W. S. 1940. Mites in the nasal passages and sinuses of dogs. Cornell Vet. 30:252-55.

Monlux, W. S., E. S. Raun, S. J. Diesch, and J. A. Hunt. 1961. Foot rot and a mucosal-type disease caused by *Chorioptes bovis.* J. Am. Vet. Med. Assoc. 138:379-81.

Muller, G. H., and R. W. Kirk. 1969. Small Animal Dermatology. W. B. Saunders, Philadelphia.

Murray, M. D. 1961. The life cycle of *Psorergates ovis* Womersley, the itch mite of sheep. Aust. J. Agric. Res. 12:965-73.

Nutting, W. B., L. C. Satterfield, and G. E. Cosgrove. 1973. *Demodex* sp. infesting tongue, esophagus, and oral cavity of *Onychomys leucogaster,* the grasshopper mouse. J. Parasitol. 59:893-96.

Olsen, O. W., and F. K. Bracken. 1950. Occurrence of the ear mite, *Raillietia auris* (Leidy, 1872) of cattle in Colorado. Vet. Med. 45:320-21.

Olsen, S. J., and H. Roth. 1947. On the mite *Cheyletiella parasitivorax,* occurring on cats, as a facultative parasite of man. J. Parasitol. 33:444-45.

Park, S. E. 1942. The cereal mite — A Pseudosarcoptes. North Am. Vet. 23:269-70.

Pound, J. M., and J. H. Oliver, Jr. 1976. Reproductive morphology of *Ornithonyssus sylviarum* (Canestrini and Fanzago) (Acari: Macronyssidae). J. Parasitol. 62:470-74.

Pullin, J. W. 1956. Preliminary observations on the incidence, effect and control of chorioptic mange in dairy cattle. Can. J. Comp. Med. Vet. Sci. 20:107-15.

Roberts, I. H., W. P. Meleney, and R. E. Pillmore. 1970. Ear-scab mites, *Psoroptes cuniculi* (Acarina: Psoroptidae), in captive mule deer. J. Parasitol. 56:1039-40.

Roberts, J. A., and J. D. Kerr. 1976. *Boophilus microplus:* Passive transfer of resistance in cattle. J. Parasitol. 62:485-89.

Schaffer, M. H., N. F. Baker, and P. C. Kennedy. 1958. Parasitism by *Cheyletiella parasitivorax.* A case report of the infestation in a female dog and its litter. Cornell Vet. 48:440-47.

Sheahan, B. J., and C. Hatch. 1975. A method for isolating large numbers of *Sarcoptes scabiei* from lesions in the ears of pigs. J. Parasitol. 61:350.

Sheather, A. L. 1915. An improved method for the detection of mange acari. J. Comp. Pathol. Ther. 28:64-66.

———. 1923. The detection of intestinal protozoa and mange parasites by a floatation technique. J. Comp. Pathol. Ther. 36:266-75.

Soulsby, E. J. L. 1968. Helminths, Arthropods and Protozoa of Domesticated Animals (Mönnig), 6th ed. Williams & Wilkins, Baltimore.

Strandtmann, R. W., and G. W. Wharton. 1958. Manual of Mesostigmatid Mites. Inst. of Acarology, Univ. of Md., College Park.

Strickland, R. K., R. R. Gerrish, T. P. Kistner, and F. E. Kellogg. 1970. The white-tailed deer, *Odocoileus virginianus,* a new host for *Psoroptes* sp. J. Parasitol. 56:1038.

Sweatman, G. K. 1956. Seasonal variations in the sites of infestation of *Chorioptes bovis,* a parasitic mite of cattle, with observations on the associated dermatitis. Can. J. Comp. Med. Vet. Sci. 20:321-36.

———. 1957. Life history, non-specificity, and revision of the genus *Chorioptes,* a parasitic mite of herbivores. Can. J. Zool. 35:641-89.

———. 1958a. Biology of *Otodectes cynotis,* the ear canker mite of carnivores. Can. J. Zool. 36:849-62.

———. 1958b. On the life history and validity of the species in *Psoroptes,* a genus of mange mites. Can. J. Zool. 36:905-9.

———. 1958c. Redescription of *Chorioptes texanus,* a parasitic mite from the ears of reindeer in the Canadian Arctic. Can. J. Zool. 36:525-28.

———. 1958d. On the population reduction of chorioptic mange mites on cattle in summer. Can. J. Zool. 36:391-97.

Theobald, A. R. 1940. Parasitic skin diseases in dogs. J. Am. Vet. Med. Assoc. 97:139-44.

Unsworth, K. 1946. Studies on the clinical and parasitologic aspects of canine demodectic mange. J. Comp. Pathol. Ther. 56:114-27.

United States Department of Agriculture. 1965. Manual on livestock ticks for animal disease eradication division personnel. USDA-ARS Publ. 91-49.

Warburton, C. 1920. Sarcoptic scabies in man and animals. Parasitology 12:265-300.

Weisbroth, S. H. 1960. Differentiation of *Dermanyssus gallinae* from *Ornithonyssus sylviarum.* Avian Dis. 4:133-37.

Wharton, G. W., and H. S. Fuller. 1952. A manual of the chiggers. Mem. Entomol. Soc. Wash., No. 4.
Whitlock, J. H. 1960. Diagnosis of Veterinary Parasitisms. Lea & Febiger, Philadelphia.

REFERENCES FOR SECTION 4

Baker, D. W. 1946. Barn itch. Parasitol. Lab., Vet. Exp. Stn., Cornell Univ.
Bishopp, F. C. 1921. *Solenopotes capillatus,* a sucking louse of cattle not heretofore known in the U.S. J. Agric. Res. 21:797-802.
Chandler, W. L. 1917. Investigations of the value of nitrobenzol as a parasiticide with notes on its use in collecting external parasites. J. Parasitol. 4:27-32.
Crystal, M. M. 1949. A descriptive study of the life history stages of the dog biting louse, *Trichodectes canis* (DeGeer) (Mallophaga:Trichodectidae). Bull. Brooklyn Entomol. Soc. 44:89-97.
Emerson, K. C. 1956. Mallophaga (chewing lice) occurring on the domestic chicken. J. Kans. Entomol. Soc. 29:63-79.
Ferris, G. F., and C. J. Stojanovich. 1951. The sucking lice. Mem. Pac. Coast Entomol. Soc., vol. 1.
Florence, L. 1921. The hog louse, *Haematopinus suis* Linné: Its biology, anatomy and histology. Cornell Univ. Agric. Exp. Stn. Mem. 51, pp. 637-743.
Hofstad, M. S., B. W. Calnek, C. F. Helmboldt, W. Malcolm Reid, H. W. Yoder (eds.) 1978. Diseases of Poultry, 7th ed. Iowa State University Press, Ames, Iowa.
Hopkins, G. H. E., and T. Clay. 1952. A Check List of the Genera and Species of Mallophaga. British Museum of Natural History, London.
Hubbard, C. A. 1947. Fleas of Western North America. Iowa State College Press, Ames.
Kellogg, V. L., and G. F. Ferris. 1915. The Anoplura and Mallophaga of North American Mammals. Leland Stanford, Jr., Univ. Pub's. (May 25)
Lapage, G. 1956. Veterinary Parasitology. Charles C Thomas, Springfield, Ill.
Lapage, G., ed. 1962. Mönnig's Veterinary Helminthology and Entomology, 5th ed. Williams & Wilkins, Baltimore.
Lukens, W. R. 1921. To detect lice on horses. J. Am. Vet. Med. Assoc. 59(n.s. 12):50.
Martin, M. 1934. Life history and habits of the pigeon louse *(Columbicola columbae* [L.]). Can. Entomol. 66:6-16.
Matthysse, J. G. 1946. Cattle lice, their biology and control. Cornell Univ. Agric. Exp. Stn. Bull. 832.
Meleney, W. P., and Ke Chung Kim. 1974. A comparative study of cattle-infesting *Haematopinus,* with redescription of *H. quadripertusus* Fahrenholz, 1916 (Anoplura: Haematopinidae). J. Parasitol. 60:507-22.
Muller, G. H., and R. W. Kirk. 1969. Small Animal Dermatology. W. B. Saunders, Philadelphia.
Murray, M. D. 1960. The ecology of lice on sheep. II. The influence of temperature and humidity on the development and hatching of the eggs of *Damalinia ovis* (L.). Aust. J. Zool. 8:357-62.
Soulsby, E. J. L. 1968. Helminths, Arthropods and Protozoa of Domesticated Animals (Mönnig), 6th ed. Williams & Wilkins, Baltimore.
Stenram, H. 1956. The ecology of *Columbicola columbae* (L.) (Mallophaga). Opusc. Entomol. (Sweden) 21:170-90.
Whitlock, J. H. 1960. Diagnosis of Veterinary Parasitisms. Lea & Febiger, Philadelphia.

REFERENCES FOR SECTION 5

Artmann, J. W. 1975. Cuterebra parasitism of an American woodcock. J. Parasitol. 61:65.
Gebauer, O. 1958. Die Dasselfliegen des Rindes und ihre Bekampfung. Parasitol. Schriftenr. No. 9.
James, M. T., and R. F. Harwood (eds.). 1969. Herms' Medical Entomology, 6th ed. Macmillan, New York.
Portschinsky, I. A. 1916. *Wohfahrtia magnifica* Schin. Sa Biologie et son rapport a l'homme et aux animaux domestiques. Bur. Entomol. Sci. Com. Min. Agric. Mem. 11(9). (In Russian)
Soulsby, E. J. L. 1968. Helminths, Arthropods and Protozoa of Domesticated Animals (Mönnig), 6th ed. Williams & Wilkins, Baltimore, pp. 356-453.
Usinger, R. L. 1966. Monograph of Cimicidae (Hemiptera-Heteroptera). Thomas Say Found. (Entomol. Soc. Am.), vol. 7.
Zumpt, F. 1965. Myiasis in Man and Animals in the Old World. Butterworth's, London.

INDEX

Acanthocephala eggs, 59, 87
Acarina, 146
Acomatacarus galli, 158
Aelurostrongylus abstrusus, 99
Air-sac mite, 154–55, 195
Alaria canis eggs, 84
Amblyomma americanum, 162, 202
Amblyomma cajennense, 162
Amblyomma maculatum, 162, 202
American dog tick, 163, 204
American screwworm fly, 229
Analgesidae family, mites, 156
Anaplasma marginale, 124, 137
Anaplasma ovis, 124
Anaticola anseris, 207
Anaticola crassicornis, 207
Anatoecus dentatus, 207
Ancylostoma caninum eggs, 75–77, 88
Ancylostoma tubaeforme eggs, 76, 98
Anoplocephala magna eggs, 25
Anoplocephala perfoliata eggs, 25
Anoplura, 205, 207
Antelope
    Cooperia oncophora eggs, 45
    Cooperia pectinata eggs, 45
    Cooperia punctata eggs, 45
    Haemonchus contortus eggs, 45–46
    Moniezia expansa eggs, 44
    Oesophagostomum columbianum eggs, 45
    Ostertagia circumcincta eggs, 45
    Ostertagia ostertagi eggs, 45
    tapeworm eggs, 44, 51
    Thysanosoma actinioides eggs, 51
    Trichostrongylus axei eggs, 45
    Trichostrongylus colubriformis eggs, 45
Applicator sticks, 163, 165, 170
Arachnida, 146
Argasidae, 147, 161
Argas persicus, 161, 200
Arthropoda, 146
Ascarid eggs. *See* host name
Ascaridia galli eggs, 113
Ascaris lumbricoides eggs, 102
Ascaris suum eggs, 58

Ascarops strongylina eggs, 63
Aspiculuris tetraptera eggs, 100
Ass. *See* Horse
Auditory canal mites, 160, 198
Auricular mange, 152, 154
Avian scabies, 150, 183–84

Babesia argentina, 124
Babesia bigemina, 124, 138
Babesia canis, 124, 138
Balantidium coli, trophozoite, 57
Banana seeds in feces, 108
Bartonella. See Haemobartonella
Bdellonyssus. See Ornithonyssus
Bear
    broad fish tapeworm eggs, 73
    Dibothriocephalus latus eggs, 73
Bedbug, 238
Beef tapeworm eggs, 107
Bighorn sheep
    coccidia, oocysts, 53
    Eimeria intricata oocysts, 53
    Eimeria ovina oocysts, 52–53
    Nematodirus spathiger eggs, 47, 88
    Psoroptes ovis, 151–52, 185–86
    scab mite, psoroptic, 151–52, 185–86
    thread-necked worm eggs, 47
Bile ducts, coccidia, oocysts, 120
Birds. *See* common name
Birds, wild
    chiggers, 157–58, 196
    feather mites, 165
    Plasmodium relictum, 127
    quill mites, 158–59
    red mites, 159, 197
    Toxoplasma gondii, 127–28, 141
Bison
    Fasciola hepatica eggs, 41
    Fascioloides magna eggs, 42
    Haemonchus contortus eggs, 45–46
    liver fluke eggs, 41
    Ostertagia ostertagi eggs, 45
    Trichostrongylus axei eggs, 45

259